"Clara's Rib is a diary of a woman from a family ravaged by tuberculosis when the death rate from ̲ ̲ ̲ ̲ ̲ vas in the range of 40%. Clara a̲ ̲ ̲ ̲ ̲ ̲ ̲ ̲ admitted to the Royal Ottawa Sa̲ ̲ ̲ ̲ ̲ ̲ ̲ 18 years respectively. John's dea̲ ̲ ̲ ̲ ̲ ̲ ̲ fragility of human life. Tuberculo̲ ̲ ̲ ̲ ̲ ̲ ̲ttending school. Over time Clara ̲ ̲ ̲ ̲ ̲, ̲vıary, and her brothers Ralph, George and Jim are admitted to the San. The disease and the surgical therapy steals the chance of having her own family and also kills her youngest brother, Billy, with TB meningitis at age four, her father, her first love and many of her closest friends. Clara finds the strength and fortitude to strive for and attain a full and complete life.

Clara's life is truly a miracle and an inspiration. One can only marvel at her inner strength. She is a hero in the true sense of the word."

Peter Jessamine MD, FRCPC
Program Director, Division of Microbiology
The Ottawa Hospital, General Campus

Dr. Jessamine's father, Dr. Alexander Gordon Jessamine, was former superintendent at the Royal Ottawa Sanatorium.

"I spent my entire eighteenth year in hospital with Clara in 1945. Clara's account of life in the San brought back vivid memories. Her detailed description captures perfectly our lives as young TB patients. She has transported me back in time to a period that evokes many feelings. I recall the sadness and fear, but also the times of great humour and laughter. There is something in this book that will touch everyone."

Myrtle Jennings Murphy, Former TB Patient

"A remarkable autobiography of the incredible and heroic struggles of a twelve-year-old with lung tuberculosis – in the time before chemotherapy. Fourteen years in and out of the sanatorium on the 'cure'. Major surgery with rib removals to collapse both lungs in efforts to close cavities, with many setbacks and overwhelming disappointments."

> "Will there ever be a drug for tuberculosis?
> Has God forsaken me?
> I need a miracle – my only chance."

Deep religious convictions.
Dedicated medical and nursing staff.
Loving romance ending in tragic death.
A second romance and marriage.
Adoption of a 2 year old son – leading to a wonderfully happy life.
She lived for her full 3 score years and ten!

She was the MIRACLE.

C. William L. Jeanes M.D.
Former Medical Director, Canadian Tuberculosis Association

"*Clara's Rib* is a touching historical read, but also a reminder of why we must not lose sight of the dangers of diseases such as TB."

"*Clara's Rib* is a lesson in perseverance and acceptance. It is, incongruously, a story with a happy ending. Despite her health challenges, Clara eventually has a family and lives into her seventies. It is also a reminder of how far we have come from the days when TB stalked this city. But the book should also sound a warning about the reemergence of tuberculosis."

Elizabeth Payne,
Ottawa Citizen

"Clara's story puts a truly human face on the formidable tuberculosis epidemic and gives us insights into Canada's Sanatorium Age. The old TB sans are disappearing, but Clara's story continues to be relevant today as an inspiration to anyone struggling with a debilitating and potentially lethal chronic illness."

Dr. Brian Graham, CEO,
Lung Association of Saskatchewan

CLARA'S RIB

A True Story of a Young girl
Growing up in a Tuberculosis Hospital

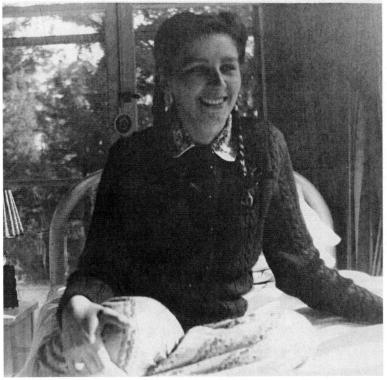

Clara Raina at the Preventorium in 1946. Nineteen years of age.

By
Clara Raina Flannigan
and Anne Raina

To Susan
Every day is beautiful.
With Best Wishes
Anne Raina

Contents

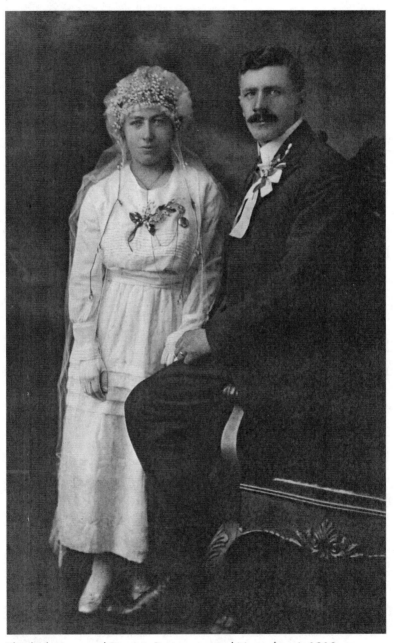

Elizabeth Hepp and Dominic Raina – married November 4, 1919 at Castor, Alberta

RAINA FAMILY

Dominic Anthony Raina
     Born November 11, 1889   Busca, Italy
     Died April 20, 1952   Kemptville, Ontario

Elizabeth Hepp
     Born September 9, 1900   Yosfvllva, Austria-Hungary
     Died October 31, 1979   Kemptville, Ontario

Dominic and Elizabeth married November 4, 1919 at Castor, Alberta

John Peter Raina
     Born August 20, 1921   Castor, Alberta
     Died December 13, 1939   Ottawa, Ontario

Mary Elizabeth Raina
     Born November 18, 1922   Castor, Alberta

Ralph Dominic Raina
     Born March 24, 1925   Castor, Alberta

Clara Kathleen Raina
     Born October 6, 1926   Hanna, Alberta
     Died May 28, 1998   Ottawa, Ontario

Louis Joseph Raina
     Born September 5, 1930   Hanna, Alberta

George Bernard Raina
     Born June 3, 1932   Hanna, Alberta
     Died September 26, 1986   Ottawa, Ontario

Dominic (Nick) Anthony Raina
    Born February 15, 1934   St. Marc de Figuery, Quebec

James Joseph Raina
    Born March 19, 1938   Ottawa, Ontario

William Paul Raina
    Born January 17, 1940   Ottawa, Ontario
    Died May 19, 1944   Ottawa, Ontario

Margaret Anne Raina
    Born December 3, 1943   Ottawa, Ontario

FOREWORD

"You have to promise me Anne," Clara urged her youngest sibling in May 1998, "that when I die you will sneak my rib into my coffin. If you don't, and it gets tossed in the garbage, just think what might happen if someone spots it in the city dump or a dog goes sniffing it out. Next thing, bulldozers and excavators will be turning the garbage dump upside down searching for the rest of the body that goes with this rib." The imagined headlines and chaos that could follow the discovery of a human rib in the local landfill caused Clara and Anne to laugh heartily.

The laughter, while genuine, was also bittersweet. Anne and Clara both knew that Anne would have to carry out this task within a few days. It was nearly time to lay both Clara and her rib to rest. On May 28, 1998, Clara's body succumbed to cancer. Her spirit, though, was unconquerable and lives on vibrantly in the memories of all who knew and loved her.

Frequently, before and after my sister Clara became ill with cancer, she had discussed her book with me and expressed her intention to bequeath it to me. I believe that only her husband Harry, her son Bill, Father Campeau, our Mother and me knew she had written this book. In all discussion we shared about the book, she gave me full permission to do whatever I wanted to do with it after her death and expressed full trust in any decisions I might make regarding any changes, whether in text, title or lay out. Two days before she died she again told me that she wanted me to have complete ownership of all her diaries, letters, taped and written versions of the book and all documents pertaining to it. I knew that previously she had submitted it to one publisher and that her hope had been to have it published. I promised her, in that final conversation about her book, that one day I would fulfill her wish.

Unfortunately, promises cannot always be kept in the time frame that we would like and life intervened. However, now the time is right.

I have not changed the text of Clara's story in any way. Her story is based on her diary entries and is completely in her own words as she wrote it. Clara wrote the Preface and the Body of this book. I have written the additional parts. During the process of creating my contributions to the book, I have sensed Clara's presence throughout every step. I feel incredibly closely united with her in this labour of love.

After considerable thought and discussion with family members and friends, and with full confidence, I did change her original title to 'Clara's Rib'. I had prayed for inspiration for an appropriate title as I typed and read and re-read her manuscript. I can see Clara's animated and enthusiastic approval. While I had always liked her original title, *Wheeze and Sneeze and Shoot the Breeze*, which came to her in a dream more than thirty years ago, it would have been more appropriate then when people had a greater awareness of tuberculosis. It still would make perfect sense after reading the book. However, unanimous initial reaction of people to the original title was that it must be a book about allergies and they would not be motivated to read it. Clara, although suffering greatly from allergies herself, would never have wanted people to think that was the subject of this book. I felt what was much more important than having her original title read, was that her inspiring story be read in its wholeness and richness. And Clara did entrust her rib to me!

The Dedication, a brief outline of *Tuberculosis, Then and Now,* and a listing of the children of Elizabeth and Dominic Raina precede the Preface.

Another change was incorporated to make the time line of the story easier for the reader to follow. After each original chapter heading, I have inserted the dates covered in that chapter and have noted the age of Clara at the time.

To offer a clearer description of some of the medical procedures and other subjects referred to in *Clara's Rib*, I have inserted footnotes numbered 1 through 15, and 18, 19, 22, and 24. Footnotes 16, 17, 20, 21, 23 and 25 were written by Clara.

All the people in the book are real. All are identified by their own names, with the exception of the following: Mrs. Thingamabob, Miss Lovely, Mrs. Good, Mrs. Waxy, Mrs. Hypo and Miss W. While the names of these characters have been changed, they are real people who interacted with Clara in the way she described.

In addition, an Afterward has been included to give a brief overview of the rest of Clara's life.

A number of people who have reviewed the book asked that I write a chapter on how I, when I was little, processed all that was happening within this large family afflicted by tuberculosis. This is a question Clara also sometimes asked me. A few of my memories and thoughts are included in a Postscript.

Anne Raina

DEDICATION

Choosing a dedication on behalf of my dear sister Clara was not a task to be taken lightly. Clara would certainly have approached her decision with great thought and prayer. There were so many people in her life who she would have wanted to honour. First and foremost would be our devoted parents, Elizabeth and Dominic Raina. She deeply loved and cherished her nine siblings with whom she shared such a close bond. Her thoughts would be filled with memories of Harold Mouré. And with love and affection she would be thinking of her adored husband Harry Flannigan and the most treasured gift in life, her son Bill. There was a multitude of friends and medical staff members who contributed to her wellbeing. All of these people were important to Clara.

But I feel that her final choice for her dedication would, in all likelihood, be three people who played a paramount role in her survival, both from the medical and spiritual perspectives. I'm taking the liberty of speaking in what I believe might be the words that Clara would wish to express.

To the 'Three Great Cs'

Doctor Duncan A. Carmichael
  for fighting to keep me alive physically against all odds.

Father Louis Campeau
  for feeding and nurturing me spiritually at all times.

Nurse Irene Clement
  for faithfully being, not only an excellent nurse, but caring, compassionate and understanding during the good times and the bad.

The three of you were my hope and my steadfast friends in my quest for survival. It was your tireless dedication that allowed me so many precious and unexpected years to share with all those who loved me and who I love so greatly.

TUBERCULOSIS (TB)
THEN AND NOW

LADY GRAY HOSPITAL
OPENS IN OTTAWA IN 1910

This Main Treatment Centre for Tuberculosis in Eastern Ontario was also known as the *Royal Ottawa Sanatorium, 'The San'.*

On February 21, 1910, the Royal Ottawa accepted its first Tuberculosis patient.

While I grew up as the youngest child in a family literally 'consumed' with tuberculosis, and the language of TB was like a second language in our home, I am aware that many people are unfamiliar with the disease called tuberculosis. For this reason, it seems relevant to provide a brief description of this insidious disease that ravaged, and continues to ravage, many families, not only in Canada, but throughout the world.

If someone had asked me as a small child what tuberculosis was, I would likely have responded that it was a disease that took my sisters and most of my brothers and my father to a big hospital and that I could hardly ever get to see them. Because nobody under 16 years of age was allowed in to visit, I would have said that when I went along with my family to visit those in the San, that I would stand alone on the lawn under the huge trees and try to find the window from which the voice calling

"Ansie" was coming. Then I would peer up at my father or whichever brother or sister was waving from the window and we would exchange some conversation. I would have said that often it was a very long time before I got to see my father or my brothers or sisters up close and that I missed them. But tuberculosis is many things.

"TB is a potentially fatal contagious disease that can affect almost any part of the body but is mainly an infection of the lungs. It is caused by a bacterial microorganism, the tubercle bacillus or Mycobacterium tuberculosis. Although TB can be treated, cured, and can be prevented if persons at risk take certain drugs, scientists have never come close to wiping it out. Few diseases have caused so much distressing illness for centuries and claimed so many lives." *Free Medical Dictionary online, April 29, 2010.*

"In 1882, the microbiologist Robert Koch discovered the tubercle bacillus, at a time when one of every seven deaths in Europe was caused by TB. Because antibiotics were unknown, the only means of controlling the spread of infection was to isolate patients in private sanatoria or hospitals limited to patients with TB – a practice that continues to this day in many countries. At the turn of the twentieth century tuberculosis was the single most common cause of death in the United States." *Free Medical Dictionary online, April 29, 2010.*

"During the first half of the 20th Century, TB was called 'consumption' or 'white plague' and it was the number one killer of Canadians. The historic menace of the 'White Plague' continued for so many centuries because people had a poor understanding of the disease and poor medical tools with which to fight it." http://www.lung.ca/tb/abouttb/what/, April 29, 2010.

According to 'An History of the Fight Against Tuberculosis in Canada', online April 29, 2010, "the 'Sanatorium Age' in Canada began in 1896, when the first institution was being built by the National Sanatorium Association of Muskoka, Ontario. The sanatoria demonstrated the value of rest, fresh air, good nutrition and isolation to prevent the spread of infection. These treatment centres specialized in the diagnosis and recovery of patients with tuberculosis. The sanatorium occupied a unique place in the tuberculosis program in North America and Western Europe and nowhere was it as well developed as in Canada."

"During the first half of the 20th century, in-patient treatment was then believed to be the only way to manage TB, and by 1938, Canada had 61 sanatoriums and special tuberculosis units in hospitals with close to 9,000 beds. This, however, was not sufficient to treat all patients suffering from tuberculosis. From 9,000 beds in 1938, the bed complement rose to a peak of 19,000 beds in 1953. Patients' average length of stay in hospital was prolonged at the time, reaching a peak of just over one year in the mid-1950s. Many patients, though, stayed at 'the San' for 3-5 years and some even longer." 'An History of the Fight Against Tuberculosis in Canada' – http://www.lung.ca/tb/tbhistory/sanatoriums/, April 29, 2010.

In the past, 'on the cure' was a very common expression in connection with tuberculosis. Persons suffering from tuberculosis were put on bed rest and it was hoped that rest, combined with good nutrition, would counter or prevent the consumptive nature of TB. Sometimes those still with active TB were sent home for periods of time 'on the cure' with the view to improvement to their health. It was also quite common for someone who had been diagnosed with tuberculosis to remain at home 'on the cure' until a bed became available in the sanatorium.

"At the end of the nineteenth century, in Ottawa, as throughout Canada, the United States, and in Europe, the mortality rate from tuberculosis was over 200 per 100,000 population." The story of the Royal Ottawa Hospital, published 1985.

In 1939, the year that Clara entered the San, there were 9,184 cases of tuberculosis recorded in Canada. That number had increased to 13,804 cases by 1952, the year that Clara left the San for the last time. Source: Tuberculosis Prevention and Control Program: Public Health Agency of Canada.

Based on Statistics Canada information, for the years 1936-40 (when our family first became infected with TB), the number of deaths in Canada was 6,265 or at a rate of 56.2 per 100,000 population. For the period 1951-55 (during which time our family was discharged from the San for the last time), the number of deaths in Canada was 2,175 or 14.6 per 100,000 population.

"Tuberculosis continues to be a major health problem worldwide. The World Health Organization (WHO) declared tuberculosis a global emergency in 1995 and warned of a specific TB emergency in Africa in 2005. It is estimated that one-third of the world's population is infected with Mycobacterium tuberculosis – the cause of TB. Approximately 9 million new cases of active TB disease develop each year, and almost 2 million persons die of the disease. Expressed otherwise, there is a new case in the world every 4 seconds and a death every 19 seconds. This makes tuberculosis a leading cause of morbidity and mortality – a fact with important implications for Canada due to international travel and immigration from high TB-incidence countries." Life and Breath: Respiratory Disease in Canada, 2007, published by the Public Health Agency of Canada and used with their permission.

"Most people who are exposed to TB bacteria do not develop TB disease as the immune system kills or effectively controls the bacteria." Life and Breath: Respiratory Disease in Canada, 2007.

According to data collected by Health Canada and available on line, there are approximately 1,600 new cases of tuberculosis reported in Canada every year. The number of cases of tuberculosis reported in Ottawa, Ontario in 2009 was 49.

March 24 is World Tuberculosis Day, held each year to mark the discovery of the cause of the disease.

No statistics can explain TB as well as Clara has done in her account of growing up with the disease.

PREFACE

During the winter of 1977 and 1978 I was in a slump, so decided to review my life. I remembered all the efforts and patience that had been devoted toward me over a number of years to culminate in my recovery from tuberculosis so long ago. Was it really worth all this work for so many people? I wondered. I was now fifty-one years old, certainly well over the hill. And I had accomplished so little in my life.

Could I be feeling sorry for myself? I pondered some more. I have always felt that self-pity and depression are our worst enemies so decided that the time had come for me to help myself. What I needed was a diversion.

I had contracted tuberculosis at age twelve and during the many years of confinement in the Sanatorium some of the nurses had suggested that I should write a book about life in the hospital but I always felt that I lacked both the talent and the education. I could not even think of a title for a book, let alone write one. Then one night I dreamed of a name and upon awakening I wrote the title down.

The dream had been forgotten for many years. Then one day I came upon some old notes and found where I had jotted down *Wheeze and Sneeze and Shoot the Breeze.* This title seemed very appropriate for my condition. Next I searched through the closets for old diaries and note books. As I read these notes, I laughed heartily and I cried freely. And I was so thankful that

I was alone in the house as I relived these experiences from the past.

Thus it was that on April 21st, 1978, my autobiography started merrily on the way to being written.

CHAPTER ONE

ALBERTA

October 6, 1926 – November 23, 1932
From Birth to Six Years, One Month

The Hanna Hospital in Alberta was the place of my birth on Wednesday, October 6th, 1926, at approximately four o'clock in the afternoon.

My homecoming took place on October the 17th, and I was baptized the same day. Father Joseph Fay performed the ceremony in St. George's Roman Catholic Church in Hanna and I was named Clara Kathleen. I was the fourth child born to Elizabeth Hepp and Dominic Raina.

Father was born in Busca, Italy, at the very foot of the Alps, on November 11th, 1889. In spite of Dad's love for his family and the beauty of the countryside, he bid farewell to his relatives in Italy when still a young man and headed for South America, where he bought a small banana plantation. Dad remained in South America for a while, returning to Italy when his father became ill. After the death of his father, he moved on to Alberta, Canada, in 1913. Father, well-educated, spoke a number of languages and believed that travel was a great education in itself.

Mother was born in Yosfvllva, Austria-Hungary on September 9th, 1900, and immigrated to Canada with her family when she was four years old. Her father, Peter Hepp, settled at Castor, Alberta, and farmed there for most of his life.

My parents met in Alberta and were married there on November 4th, 1919.

The first six years of my life were spent living on a farm at Dowling, Alberta, and those were very happy years. I loved my parents dearly and the days were filled with happy childhood memories.

Weather permitting, my days would begin by going outside in search of Father. Dad always seemed so pleased and I can still remember the happy expression on his face the day he said "My little girl always comes to say good morning to her daddy." I think that those morning greetings will always be the fondest memories that I have of my Father.

There were always interesting things to do with my sister and brothers or by myself. We loved to find the first crocuses in the spring – and to hunt for crows' nests and to catch gophers. There was a bounty for gopher tails and crows' eggs which would provide us children with a few pennies.

During the summer I would play in the sand for hours at a time as the sand always felt so warm and comfortable. Ralph would let me play with his Sandy Andy which was a favourite toy in the sand pile. Then there was an occasional barefoot walk through fresh cow chips which could be fun after a warm rain.

We also enjoyed riding horseback on Nellie, the one horse that was kept inside the stable and ready for riding at a moment's notice. I must not forget to mention Rushlight, the Shetland pony. However, I do not remember this pony as ever rushing, but think of him as an old, tired-out pet that we pampered and loved.

When our brother Louis was born in 1930, I was evicted from my crib and was happy to be able to share a double bed with my sister. Mary was nearly four years older than I was and she was our writer, poet and story teller. After we were in bed at night Mary would tell me numerous fairy tales which provided me with an endless amount of joy and excitement. When her supply of known stories was exhausted and I was still begging for more, Mary would carry right on by inventing stories of her own. Mary's stories were even more exciting than the storybook tales as hers usually carried a certain amount of mystery to them. I might be left for minutes guessing what was found at the end of a trail before I was given the punch line.

Mary's imagination was always wide awake and she tells of feeding me eggshells when I was small as she had hoped that this would enable me to lay eggs. Ironically, more eggs were something that Alberta was not in need of at that time. Surprisingly, Mary and I had very few fights and she was really a good big sister – and I was a good little sister as I believed all of her stories as the gospel truth. If I ever did doubt any of her tales and planned to ask Mother, Mary always had a good reason why I should not be asking questions.

Mary even convinced me that she and my brother John had worked for a gum company and that their chore was to chew the gum before it was packaged so it would be of the right consistency when it was sold. She said that all the children that were employed wore special hats as they sat around chewing gum. Just to think of John and Mary chewing gum all day made me a little envious of their good fortune. Once again I was warned that I must never speak about their exciting occupation as people would cease to buy gum if they knew that it had been already chewed before reaching the store shelves.

The Christmas Concerts were one of the biggest events of the year and were usually enjoyed by every member of the family. I remember one year in particular when I was eagerly awaiting the school concert and then I came down with a bad cold. Mother stayed home with me, and Dad took the three older children to the concert by horse and sleigh. Mother must have been disappointed when we bid the party-goers good-bye but she never showed it as she played games with me that evening. I had my doll and we played house – then Mother took out some candies that she had hidden away for Christmas and we had our own party. As we partied Mother remarked that she was sure we were having more fun than the ones at the concert were having. I really do believe that I had more fun but Mother must have been very disappointed as she seldom got out in those days. That evening is the fondest memory that I have of my Mother from the days of my childhood and I think it was a good example of what Christmas is really all about.

We were aware of our parents' great love for us in spite of Dad's strictness and we also knew that we never could get away with any nonsense. "Get Down On Your Knees" was Dad's favourite form of punishment. However, if the offence was of a serious nature, the punishment would be more severe and we would have to place our hands underneath our knees and kneel on them for a while. I remember committing one serious offence when about four years old. Mary wondered how Dad would react if one of us children would call him Dominic and I was the candidate elected for this experiment. Thus, one morning, while Dad sat at his desk, I greeted him in this manner "Good morning Dominic, how are you?" I soon found out how Dad was and it wasn't happy. I was told to kneel down and put my hands underneath my knees. As I knelt, I was given a lengthy lecture about children having respect for their parents and never to address them by their first name. The entire time that I was down on my knees I could see Mary's eyes on me and they convinced me that it would indeed be very foolish to tell Dad that she had coached me for the Good Morning Dominic

Caper. That was the first and last time that I remember any of the Raina children calling our father Dominic.

Our brother George was born in June of 1932 and he was the sixth child in our family. In September of that year I started to school and was happy to be tagging along with John, Mary and Ralph. We walked to the Wiese School which was about a mile and a half from home. I loved school and I loved the West so it was a sad day when our parents decided to leave Alberta in the fall of that year.

When the final arrangements for our departure were completed, it was agreed that Mary, Ralph and I would go to Castor and spend a few days with our Grandmother Hepp while John remained at home to help with the auction sale. Right from the beginning things did not go too well between my Grandmother and me and I feel that I never ranked as one of her favourite grandchildren. Gramma was so full of enthusiasm when she took us to see my first movie ever, a Charlie Chaplin film. Even though the show was good I slept through most of it, much to the disappointment of my Grandmother.

Next came the episode with the lights. We still used coal oil lamps on the farm but Grandmother had electricity and that magic chain that turned the light on and off really fascinated us, especially Mary. That ever-active mind of hers decided to take advantage of the cold that I was coming down with and after we were in bed that night the fun began. Mary had me expertly trained and when she said "Cough" on went the light, then again "Cough" and off went the light. How we marvelled at the speed at which a room could constantly be changed from total darkness into light. Apart from our enchantment with electricity, all was not total happiness as Mary's nearly ten-year-old shoulders were weighted down with other problems. Gramma did not have indoor plumbing and a trip outdoors in the middle of the night did not appeal to us. Oh yes, there was a small chamber potty underneath the bed, but that was part of our problem. The magic chain had kept us awake, and the excitement had caused us to reach underneath the bed several times and now the chamber potty runneth over and our bladders could not hold out until morning. To go outside or to empty the chamber potty meant a trip downstairs and we feared the lady that was staying with Gramma. However, I could always rely on my older sister to think of a solution and once again she did not fail me. Silently, she crept to the window and pried it open. Then the overflowing container was cautiously carried and hastily dumped on the ground below, facing a street in Castor. Gramma never said anything but to this day I still wonder if Gramma knew what caused that large yellow patch in the snow at the front of her house.

My cold was worse when we went downstairs the next morning but Grandmother showed no sympathy while telling me to quit the coughing as she knew it was only an act. Mrs. Thingamabob who lived with Gramma had already reported her findings – every time that I had coughed, she had heard the light chain.

After the auction sale, Mother came to Castor with the rest of the children. Then John, Mary and Ralph were allowed to go and visit our relatives in the country for a few days. They were the Muhlbeier family, the Hepps and the Justs. By this time Gramma was convinced that I really did have a cold so I could not accompany the older children, much to my disappointment. Then Gramma tried to treat my cold with hot onion tea but I gagged and refused to drink it. Needless to say, I was not endearing myself to my loving Grandmother.

On November 23rd, 1932, we boarded the train in Alberta and headed for our new destination. Shortly after the train pulled away from the station another passenger became aware of my constant coughing and then this kindly lady came over and gave me some white peppermint candies to suck on. No sooner had the lady departed when Mary reminded me about Snow White and the poisoned apple. Then she warned me this lady might be a witch in disguise and the candies could be poisoned. Nevertheless I ate the candies, but with caution and a great deal of apprehension.

My cold was actually the whooping cough that hung on for a long time and I did not return to school until the following September.

Thus ended the first years of my life, when we left the Province of Alberta. Six years and one month of a happy childhood and a treasure of wonderful memories.

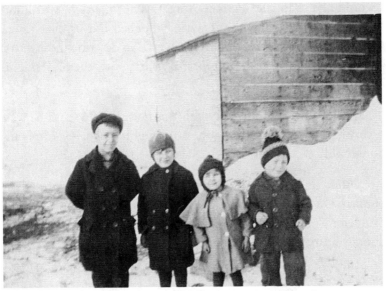

Left to Right: John, Mary, Clara and Ralph Raina, Dowling, Alberta

CHAPTER TWO

PLEASE ALLOW ME TO FORGET

November 1932 to April 1937
From Six Years, One Month to Ten Years, Six Months

From November 1932 to April 1937 is a time in my life that I would like to forget. Perhaps 'forget' is not the right word but I do not like speaking about what happened during that time. First of all I cannot find the proper words to describe those years and, secondly, if I did attempt to write about them, I might become too emotional.

Our brother, Dominic (Nick), was born in 1934 and he was a very sweet and lovable baby, so brought much joy into our household.

Otherwise, our family life was filled with a great deal of sorrow and we all wished to escape from the source of our problems. Thus it was with joy and relief that we left the land of doom on April 1st, 1937, and headed for Ottawa, penniless.

CHAPTER THREE

ONTARIO

April 1937 – September 1939
From Ten and One Half Years to Twelve Years, Eleven
Months

I was ten and a half years old when we arrived in Ottawa in the month of April 1937. After spending two months in the city, we moved out on Highway 31, about three miles from Ottawa. Once again our lives became more secure and I enjoyed going to Ellwood School and later to St. Thomas Aquinas School at Billings Bridge.[1]

Times were hard and each member of the family had to do their share of work. Dad and Mother milked cows for a dairy farmer near home and for their work they received free rent and milk. John worked full time on a dairy farm and some of the other children did various chores for the local gardeners. We picked strawberries for two cents a quart and raspberries for three cents a quart. We also weeded gardens and picked beans

---

1 Billings Bridge, the area where we lived, was a small village surrounded mainly by agricultural land in Gloucester Township. The home on the farm that we rented was eventually demolished when the current Alta Vista Public School was built on Randall Avenue. Its doors opened in April 1949. Billings Bridge was annexed by the City of Ottawa in 1950. On Bank Street, the Billings Bridge Shopping Plaza constructed in the 1950s marked a definite shift from rural life to a more commercial one.

and potatoes in harvest time. The money that we earned was turned over to our parents.

I always enjoyed picking berries so considered this occupation more of a pleasure than it was work. As for picking potatoes, that was one job that I positively loathed. The weather was usually cold and damp at that time of the year and I would be chilled to the bone as I gathered up those moist potatoes. Most children under fourteen would receive twenty-five cents a day and it was customary to work until dusk. I had to go picking potatoes on my twelfth birthday and I really felt sorry for myself. I always hated missing school for any reason and, above all things, having to miss to pick potatoes on this all-important day. Some of the boys from our classroom were also there picking potatoes but I think they preferred this to going to school. When we arrived home after dark there was a chocolate cake waiting for us that Mother had baked for my birthday.

Another brother was born in 1938 and we commented to Mother that she seemed to enjoy Jimmy so much that one would think he was her first child. Mother then explained to us children that no matter how large the family is, parents always have enough love for each child and that no one is ever loved less because there are several children.

We liked Ontario and everything seemed to be falling into place. The children were doing well in school. The boys had become altar boys and we went to church regularly. Father Lee devoted a great deal of time to choir practice and tested each pupil individually for singing abilities. I did my utmost to convince Father Lee that I could not sing but my protests were in vain and I had to give him a sample of my musical abilities. When I stood up in class and opened my mouth to sing my emotions could have better been expressed if I had just brayed as that was exactly how I felt. I had often tried my voice for singing when alone in some back field at home and the sound that emerged was no sound that anyone would wish to hear in church.

When the testing was completed, we were classified – some had very good voices, some should not sing alone but could do very well in a choir – the remaining ones should refrain from ever singing. I was not surprised to learn that I had made the last category. Father Lee then expressed his disappointment at the Raina family's lack of ability to sing, because we were among his best church-goers. After that, whenever Father Lee had choir practice, the few 'non-singers' would go into another classroom and do school work. For some this was an opportunity to chew up the large supply of bubblegum that they would bring along with them.

Early in June of 1939 Ralph contracted scarlet fever and we were under quarantine for several weeks. John had a lingering cough and after x-rays and tests it was confirmed that he was suffering from tuberculosis of the lungs. He was instructed to remain in bed at home until there was a place available for him in the Royal Ottawa Sanatorium.

Ralph had barely recovered from scarlet fever when Mary became ill with the red measles. Within a few days, all eight children were in bed with the measles and most of us were quite ill so our parents were kept busy day and night caring for us. John was already quite sick and now with this additional illness, things did not look good and Mother worried a great deal over her eldest son.

Several of us were complaining of chest pains while slowly recovering from the measles but in spite of the persistent pains we were up and about and attended school on opening day in September. I always loved the outdoors and only stayed inside when necessary. And after having the measles I still loved the outdoors as much as ever but I would sit on the steps instead of playing or going for walks. One day as I sat outside I overheard Mother telling Dad that she was sure there was something wrong with me as she had seen me sitting on the steps on two different occasions that day and that I never sat down when I was outside. As for the chest pains, we tried to convince ourselves and each other that they were caused from eating apples that were still too green.

In the meantime we were all waiting to have x-rays since it was discovered that John had tuberculosis.

CHAPTER FOUR

COME HERE
LITTLE CHILDREN TO SUFFER

September 1939 – March 2, 1940
Twelve Years, Eleven Months to Thirteen Years, Five Months

In the early part of September 1939, John was admitted into the Whitney Building of the Royal Ottawa Sanatorium ('The San') on Carling Avenue.

The rest of the family went for chest x-rays and we soon learned that those 'green apple pains' were actually pleurisy pains as the result of having had the measles.[2]

Ralph, George and I would have to quit school and go 'on the cure'. George was to remain in bed at home for three months and then go back to the Sanatorium for another chest x-ray. Ralph was admitted into the Children's Preventorium (the Pre) building at the Royal Ottawa San. I was to remain at home until we received further word from the Sanatorium. This

---

2 "Pleurisy is the inflammation of the pleura, the linings surrounding the lungs. Pleurisy is frequently associated with the accumulation of extra fluid in the space between the two layers of pleura. The chest pain of pleurisy is very distinctive. It is usually sharp and aggravated by breathing. The doctor can often hear the friction that is generated by the rubbing of the two inflamed layers of pleura with each breath. With large amounts of pleural fluid there can be decreased breath sounds and the chest is dull sounding when the doctor drums on it. Removal of pleural fluid with a needle and syringe (aspiration) is key in diagnosing the cause of pleurisy." http://www.medterms.com/script/main/art.asp?articlekey=4948, 04/05/2010.

really upset me and I emphatically protested that I was not too sick to go to school.

My protests were all in vain as word came for me to enter the Sanatorium on Monday, September 25th, 1939. I was in a nasty mood and wallowing in self-pity as I prepared to leave for the hospital. My brother Jimmy, who was eighteen months old at the time, came and tugged at my skirt and wanted me to pick him up but I just pushed him aside. Mother suggested that I might feel better if I held Jimmy for a few minutes as I would not be seeing him for a while and would probably miss him. I took Mother's advice and held our delightful little brother and discovered that I was in a much better mood when I left home for the hospital. Mother always wanted us to be at peace with each other and with ourselves before leaving the house to go anywhere.

I was also admitted into the Preventorium and was in a room alone which was at the opposite end of the building from where Ralph was. We could see from one end of the place right to the other end as the upper half of the rooms were separated with large glass windows.

Shortly after I was admitted, one of the girls from on the balcony came in to get acquainted. Penny was also twelve years old and was a large, hefty girl for her age. We had just begun speaking when my supper was brought in and Penny lost no time in informing me that we had to eat all of the food on our tray and, with emphasis, she said that also meant the entire baked potato. After my indoctrination Penny left the room.

It was with great difficulty that I managed to clean up the tray and just as I finished the last mouthful I could hear someone chuckling close by. I turned around to check where the laughter was coming from and there stood Penny watching me through the glass window that separated us. Then she returned to inform me that it was not true that we had to eat all the food that was on our tray. When the nurse returned she remarked, "You must have been very hungry." If she had only known the truth!

During the years that followed I witnessed many jokes that were played on new patients. A good sense of humour was necessary in order to survive the many months or years that were spent in the Sanatorium at that time.

A few days after I was admitted, the girls were moved inside from the unheated balcony where they had spent the summer and I now shared a room with Penny and two other girls. I soon learned that Penny never missed an opportunity for a joke or a trick and I often wondered what might have happened if Penny and my sister Mary had ever gotten together as they both used their imagination to the fullest.

When I entered the Sanatorium the regular night nurse had just left for a month of holidays. Every day Penny would tell me about Miss Lovely, she was a real Mona Lisa. According to Penny, Miss Lovely possessed great beauty and charm. Her hair was blond and curly, she had a cute little nose, she was young, her figure was streamlined, her legs were utterly beautiful and she always wore high-heeled shoes on duty. How could anyone be so beautiful and not be a movie star, I wondered.

The day finally arrived for Miss Lovely to return and Penny expressed her excitement many times. Now it was just past 7 p.m. and the nurse would soon enter to take our temperatures.

Then the door opened and Miss Lovely walked in, and the next few minutes were complete torture and I experienced one of the most embarrassing times in my life. Penny's face remained completely placid the entire time as she inquired, "Did you have a nice time *Miss Lovely?* It is so nice to have you back *Miss Lovely.*" Penny wanted me to know that there was no mistake, that this was indeed the Miss Lovely whom she had been telling me about. However, there was one thing wrong. When the door opened, it was not Mona Lisa who entered.

This nurse was a middle-aged scarecrow, her hair was messy and her nurse's cap was askew on her head. She had a figure like a sack of potatoes and her feet were being dragged across the floor inside a pair of flat, solid black shoes. All of this was just too much for me and I giggled and giggled as my reddened face burned with embarrassment. The harder I tried to stop, the more I giggled. I just could not decide which was the funniest, Miss Lovely or Penny's placid face. I was so ashamed of myself.

When Miss Lovely took my temperature and pulse my stomach was shaking and my bed was shaking and the thermometer was rattling inside my mouth as it clicked against my teeth. Then Miss Lovely spoke to me for the first time and I shall never forget these words. "My, but you are a bold little girl. You have been giggling ever since I walked into this room." And, as she spoke, her spittle splattered all over my face. As I continued to giggle, some very unpleasant thoughts were going through my mind. I wondered if they would report this kind of behaviour to my parents. If they did, Dad would not be pleased.

In 1939 the Sanatorium consisted of three buildings for tubercular patients. This was the only malady treated there at that time. The Whitney Building housed the most seriously ill patients. The Perley Building had a dining room and other facilities for the patients who were able to be up and about. The Preventorium Building cared for the children and some teenagers. In later years the age limit went up for girls and there even was an occasional married woman among the patients in the Pre.

There was also a residential building for the doctors, nurses, and other employees. The laundry building was nestled among the trees at the rear of the premises. The Workshop was situated close to the Whitney and Perley Buildings, thus making it easily accessible for brief encounters among the patients.

Dr. Duncan A. Carmichael was the Superintendent of the Sanatorium and he was a very fine and dedicated man. Dr. Lehman was second in command and he too was a good doctor but his personality was very different from that of Doctor Carmichael. Both of these doctors were to play very important roles in my life during the following years.

Miss Irene Ann Clement was the head nurse at the Preventorium and was the right person for this position. She was as dedicated as Dr. Carmichael was and both were interested in helping as many patients as possible to recover from tuberculosis. During the following years, Miss Clement became like a second mother and Doctor Carmichael was like a second father and I loved them both dearly.

In 1939 the treatment or 'cure' for TB consisted mainly of bed rest and fresh air. The windows were kept wide open both day and night.

Some patients received pneumothorax, which temporarily collapsed the diseased lung for as long as it required for it to heal. For a few others who were unable to take pneumothorax, there was the more drastic thoracoplasty surgery which consisted of removing several ribs so the diseased portion of a lung could be permanently collapsed.

Ralph and I both made good progress as we only had pleurisy and before long we were allowed to go downstairs to the dining room for our meals.

Meanwhile, over at the Whitney, things were not going well with our brother John. There were not any feasible treatments that could be used in his case, other than bed rest and fresh air.

As bodies rested, minds were ever active, especially Penny's. One night after 'lights out' Penny thought that it was time we had a little excitement so she removed a wheel from her bed. Then she rushed up to the desk to tell Miss Lovely about the wheel that had suddenly fallen off her bed. Miss Lovely was already comfortably settled in her recliner, her nurse's cap and false teeth were removed and she was snoring, although she always denied ever sleeping while on duty. The false teeth were hastily mouthed and then Miss Lovely came and replaced the wheel as we lay giggling under our covers while pretending that we were asleep.

It was much later that night and still no one was able to sleep when Penny suddenly jumped out of bed and decided it was time for an encore. The snoring Miss Lovely was again disturbed and her false teeth were hastily mouthed. Once again the rest of us lay snickering under our covers while Miss Lovely panted and sputtered while replacing the wheel. She told Penny that her bed was unsafe and another bed would have to be found for her to sleep in. We could hear Penny vehemently protesting as she was led away to sleep in the only other vacant bed in the Preventorium. The vacant bed was a crib and we were able to peek at the whole performance through the glass windows that separated the upper portions of the rooms. Penny's face looked very sober whenever we waved to her as she lay all curled up in the crib and we giggled for most of the night.

Penny wasn't the only one with an active imagination. One day this lady came over to the Pre and she told us about a conversation that had taken place a few days earlier between her and Ralph in the Workshop. She had inquired about the inscription over the door at the Preventorium as she had not been able to get close enough to read it.   "Oh, that just says '*Come Here Little Children to Suffer*'" replied Ralph, as he walked away. Ralph's answer had really mystified this lady until she came over to the Preventorium and read the inscription for herself. It said, "Red Cross Preventorium, Suffer Little Children to Come Unto Me."

Ralph and I continued to improve and were able to enjoy more activities.   Meanwhile, John's condition was steadily worsening. Finally one day Dr. Lehman allowed Ralph and me to join our sister and brothers to visit John in his room at the Whitney Building. We were all pleased to see each other but John looked so ill and was so thin. Yet he insisted that he felt fine and told us not to worry. However, we were sad and upset after we left John's room and I didn't sleep too well that night.

Some of the patients in the Preventorium received 'Sunlamp' treatments and I was among the ones being treated. We would start off with a few minutes and gradually work up to twenty minutes front and back every second day. It was while I was under the lamp on December 13th that the nurse came in to inform me that my parents were waiting downstairs and that I was to join them and Ralph as soon as the treatment was finished and I was dressed. As it was not a visiting day I immediately thought "John must be dead," and I did not want it to be so – I wanted a miracle. However, there was no miracle and John had died earlier that morning at the age of eighteen. Gone was our oldest brother who used to make swings for us. John who used to make Parcheesi games, bingo games and many other games that we couldn't afford to buy. John, who used to laugh so heartily at Mary's poetry and at Ralph's comical antics.

Ralph and I were not allowed to go home to John's wake or funeral as Doctor Lehman feared that we would catch cold and have a setback.

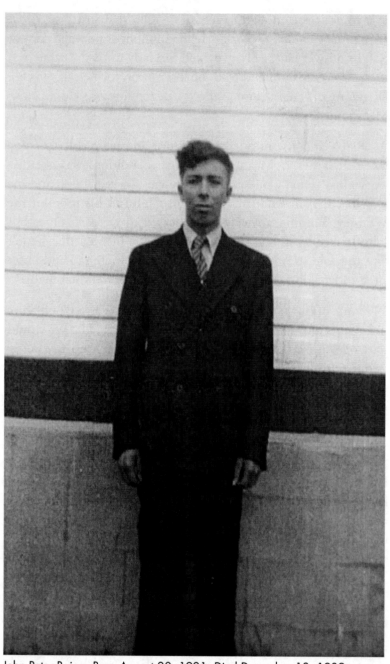

John Peter Raina, Born August 20, 1921; Died December 13, 1939.

Nov. 18, 1939

Dear Brother & Sister,

I took a notion to write, I am not so sleepy to-night. How are you both. I still have the terrible temperature but I have no pains or aches and I feel real good. Thanks a lot for the purse. Do not think my writing is shaky because I am sick. It is because I usually put my pad on a book and I can't get up to get the book. Thank you for the mass and for praying for me. Do not worry about me. I hope you can come and see me soon. I am glad Lena could go downstairs to mass. I will try to write soon

Your brother
John

Letter written to his brother and sister, Ralph and Clara, by John Raina, dated Nov. 18, 1939, when he was in the San dying of tuberculosis.

Nov. 25 1939

Dear Brother and Sister

Just a short letter to let you know I am feeling fine. When I can get something hard to put my pad on I will write better. Do you feed your Gold-fish, I know they will feed for them. I thank you both for praying for me. My Temp. was down to-day. It was 99.1 at noon and 102.2 to-night. I saw some of the snow.
I'll write again

Your Brother
John

Letter written to Clara and Ralph by John Raina, dated November 25, 1939, eighteen days before he died.

Dr. Carmichael had surgery in 1939 and Doctor Lehman was in charge during his absence. It was during this time that Doctor Lehman noticed the numerous warts that I had on my hands and arms and he tried to charm them away. He gave me a penny with the instructions that I was to count my warts every evening and then sleep with the penny beneath my pillow. I followed the good doctor's orders but I still had my warts – and I still had his penny.

After the New Year of 1940, Ralph and I were allowed to take daily walks down the street and this was referred to as 'exercise'. A patient usually began on ten minutes' exercise once or twice a day and could work up to as long as an hour twice daily – all depending on the condition of the patient.

On January 17th, 1940, one month and four days after our brother John died, Mother gave birth to another son, William Paul.

Ralph and I were both discharged from the Sanatorium on March 2nd, 1940. It was so good to be back home with our parents, sister and brothers and to meet our dear little brother Billy for the first time.

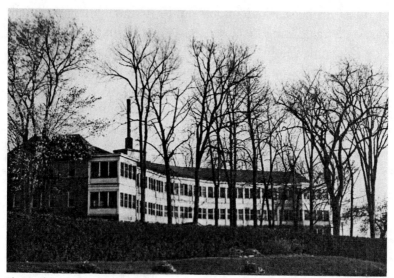

The Perley Memorial Building.

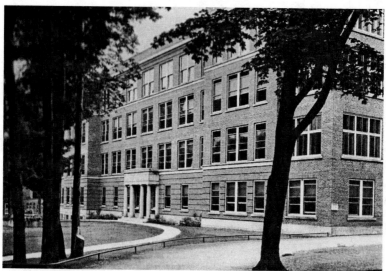

The Whitney Building, c. 1933.

CHAPTER FIVE

BACK TO SCHOOL

March 3, 1940 – June 30, 1941
Thirteen Years, Five Months – Fourteen Years, Eight Months

The following week was a time of great excitement as I was back in school again. However, there were a couple of things that were cause for concern. It was now March and I had been away from school since the early part of September. Would I get my year and be promoted with the rest of the class?

And I still had numerous warts on my hands and arms and would be embarrassed whenever anyone would make a comment about them. I usually wore long sleeves and would try to hide the warts as much as possible. Mother suggested that I should make a Novena to St. Anne so I decided to give it a try even though I wasn't expecting a miracle.[3] However, I was in for a pleasant surprise. All of my warts were smaller by the fifth or sixth day and were almost totally gone by the ninth and last day of the novena. I have read that warts sometimes will disappear very suddenly for no apparent reason but nevertheless I have had great faith in St. Anne since that time.

The day finally arrived when we received our report cards and I was promoted into grade eight with honours. Things were looking up again and life was beautiful.

---

3   In the Roman Catholic Church, a Novena is a recitation, on nine consecutive days, of prayers and devotions for a special purpose.

I had walked to Mass and received Holy Communion every morning during the month of May and God must have heard all of my prayers.

When school re-opened in September 1940 I was in grade eight and I was beginning to think of high school and about my future. I dreamed of going to the Immaculata High School in Ottawa. Later on when I would join the working force I would be very cautious with my money so I could afford to buy a riding horse of my own. I had always loved horses and every time that I went to the Winter Fair I think that mentally I went over each hurdle with all of the competitors. Some day I would have a riding pony. I continued to dream.

I still had to report to the Sanatorium regularly for x-rays and on one occasion Doctor Jeffrey had a long conversation with me. He explained that I was at a very dangerous age: that they find many girls who have had tuberculosis before reaching the age of puberty have great difficulty getting through this stage in their lives without having a relapse and once again becoming ill with TB. Thus, he cautioned me. If my parents show concern and do not think that I am well – or if I begin to lose weight – or if I get a cold that hangs on, then I am to return immediately for a checkup and not wait for the usual time to elapse between x-rays.

I never did tell my parents what the doctor had told me. Why worry them?

I still loved outdoor activities as much as ever. Mother would say that the worst problem she had with me as a child was trying to keep me indoors when I had a cold. Some of us also gave Mother a hard time when she tried to keep us home from church when we were ill. We did not want to commit a Mortal Sin and our conscience could not accept a severe cold as sufficient reason for missing Mass.

When winter arrived in 1940 it brought with it one cold after another and Sister St. Mildred was ever ready with her bottle of cod liver oil. The students who took cod liver oil kept a spoon in their desk in which to receive their daily oil. Nearly every time that I coughed Sister would say "Clara, I think that you should go and take an extra spoon of cod liver oil."

As the winter progressed and spring of 1941 arrived, I continued to have colds. My parents were worried. And Sister St. Mildred continued to push her cod liver oil. I was even given bottles to take home for weekend medication. If I wasn't smelling cod liver oil, I was burping it. I was beginning to wonder if Purgatory might actually be a cave full of cod liver oil that we would have to consume before we would be allowed into heaven and that Sister St. Mildred would be appointed as keeper of the cave.[4]

Strenuous activities made me cough so Sister St. Mildred always called me aside whenever she saw me skipping rope or playing ball. My parents wanted me to eat more lunch at noon and not rush back to school to play ball. Inwardly I suspected that all was not well as I was losing weight and I could not forget all those grim warnings that I had received from Dr. Jeffrey at my previous checkup.

Finally on May 13th I went to the Sanatorium for an x-ray and was told to return in one week for the results.

May the 20th dawned bright and beautiful and I enjoyed walking the half mile or so to attend seven o'clock Mass and to receive Holy Communion. I had gone to Mass every morning so far that month and intended to go for the remainder of May,

---

4   "The Catechism of the Catholic Church defines Purgatory as a "purification, so as to achieve the holiness necessary to enter the joy of heaven," which is experienced by those "who die in God's grace and friendship, but still imperfectly purified" (CCC 1030). http://www.catholic.com/library/Purgatory.asp, 23/08/2010.

just as I had done the previous year. After Mass I returned home for breakfast and then headed to school. This was all done in haste so I would have time to play ball before the bell rang at nine.

During morning class I thought of what lay ahead and carefully made my plans for the remainder of the day.

I rushed home at noon and ate hastily. Then I changed my clothes and hurried back to school so I could play ball. And once again Sister St. Mildred called me away from the ball game. She wanted to know why I was at school when I had to go for my medical report. I explained that there was time to play ball as I did not have to be at the Sanatorium before two o'clock. Sister said all the nuns were worried over me as they did not think that I looked well. She also mentioned that she had seen me at Mass every morning, which was nice, but that she felt it might be wiser if I remained in bed longer and rested until it was time to get ready for school.

As I prepared to leave, Sister once again expressed her fears as to what the results of my x-ray might be and assured me of her prayers.

When I arrived at the Sanatorium Dr. Lehman called me into his office and stuck a thermometer into my mouth and while my temperature was being taken he listened to my chest.

From the look on his face I knew that all was not well and, as the expression goes, my heart sank right down into my shoes. It was a horrible sensation and I felt numb. The day no longer seemed sunny and beautiful and I knew the bomb was about to fall.

Then Doctor Lehman spoke. He said there were some spots on my left lung and I would have to go back 'on the cure'. There were not any beds available in the Sanatorium so I was to remain in bed at home for one month. Then I would return for another x-ray and if there wasn't any improvement they would re-admit me into the Sanatorium.

Many thoughts raced through my mind as I slowly wended my way home. How can I tell my parents the dreadful news? What about school? How can I get my grade eight this year? The world can fall apart so fast.

A few weeks later there was one day of rejoicing. Louis came home from school and he presented me with my grade eight certificate. The Inspector had been at school and it was decided that my year's work was worthy of the diploma.

Now all I had to do was to get well and I would be off to High School.

I did not realize that when I walked out of the classroom on May 20th, 1941, that it was my final exit as a student. All those dreams that I had a few months earlier would never come true. There would be no Immaculata High School for me. Nor would there ever be a riding horse. And I never would become a member of the working force. As gloomy as the world seemed that day, it was fortunate that I couldn't see into the future!

CHAPTER SIX

RETURN TO THE SANATORIUM

July 5, 1941 – November 23, 1943
Fourteen Years, Nine Months – Seventeen Years, One Month

July 5th, 1941

I was readmitted into the Preventorium. Doctors Carmichael and Lehman, and Miss Clement were still there and it was nice seeing their familiar faces. However, I did miss my parents and family very much during those first days back in the Sanatorium.

I can't remember the contents of the first letter that I wrote home but I will never forget Ralph's comments when he came to visit me. "Imagine you saying that it is just like being in a morgue. Now you can guess what that did to Mother. Please don't ever write another letter like that again." I really did feel sorry for causing my Mother so much pain. After that I tried to spare my parents' feelings and usually kept the bad news to myself for as long as possible, or until a doctor or a nurse would pass this information on to my family.

Christmas Day 1941

We were allowed to go home for the day and I was so happy to see all the family again. Billy didn't recognize me at first and

I felt sad inside but we were quickly reacquainted. Jimmy and Billy are very good friends and are a couple of cute little guys.

February 1942

I have been on a routine of bed rest and only allowed up for bathroom privileges since being admitted. Dr. Carmichael said that in spite of all the rest, my x-ray has not shown much improvement. And perhaps I am one of those people who heal better when moving around more so he is allowing me to go downstairs to the dining room for one meal daily. My two roommates, Ethel and Teresa were also ordered up for their meals so there was a great deal of excitement in our room early today.

May 1942

Ethel, Teresa and I were put on fifteen minutes of walking exercise so now we can walk along Carling Avenue and go into the stores. We are three very happy and excited girls. Doctor Carmichael said that my x-ray still isn't showing much improvement but my sedimentation rate is very good so that was his reason for allowing me to go on exercise.[5]

Shortly after I returned to the San last July I got large abscesses underneath my arms and these continued for several months. At first Doctor Carmichael thought they were tubercular but after extensive lab work only a staphylococcus infection could be found. Doctor Carmichael suggested that I should check the Bible and see if I had as many abscesses as Job had boils.

After Easter we were moved out on the balcony for the summer months and we are enjoying it very much. We can

---

5 "A sedimentation rate or 'sed rate' is a blood test that detects and is used to monitor inflammation activity. It is measured by recording the rate at which red blood cells (RBCs) sediment in a tube over time. It increases (the RBCs sediment faster) with more inflammation." http://www.medterms.com/script/main/art.asp?articlekey=5215, 29/04/2010.

watch all the traffic going by on Carling Avenue. Another source of happiness is being able to hear the juke box being played across the street when the door is open during warm weather season. We often fall asleep at night while listening to *Oh Daddy You Aught To Get The Best For Me* and numerous other tunes.

July 1, 1942

Dr. Carmichael gave Mary permission to take me out for supper and to a movie which I enjoyed very much.

Later in July 1942

Ethel, Teresa and I decided to go and visit St. Francis Church on Wellington Street while on exercise. We felt in need of a little spiritual uplifting and I think that we feel better now that we have spoken to Our Lord in church.

Still Summer 1942

The doctor had told me that if all my tests were satisfactory that I would be going home when Ethel and Teresa were discharged. However, my sedimentation went up to fourteen and I came down with the mumps. Ethel and Teresa were discharged. When Dr. Carmichael spoke about my x-ray he did not sound optimistic nor did he mention the word 'home'. Now that I have recovered from the mumps I am all alone on my walks. I miss my two roommates ever so much.

Later that Summer 1942

Mother knows how much I enjoy fresh corn on the cob so she prepared a real feast for us girls here on the balcony. Mom fried a young chicken. Then she wrapped the meat and cooked corn in several layers of waxed paper, then newspaper. When all was ready, my brother Louis hopped on his bicycle and brought the food all the way to the Sanatorium from our home at Billings

Bridge. Newspaper is great for holding the heat and the food was deliciously hot when we ate it. There have been numerous occasions since becoming ill when I have thanked God for my wonderful family.

October 1942

This has been a happy month. I was allowed to go home for a day to celebrate my 16th birthday. Another pleasant occasion was the day Dr. Carmichael took several of the patients for a drive in his car. He was a lively and comical commentator as we drove along. After all this, I was given another half day off to go uptown with Mary and Ralph. They took me shopping for a pair of galoshes. Then we went to a movie and out to supper.

Early November 1942

The time is rapidly approaching for another checkup and my family thinks that I will soon be home for good. I was also thinking that I would be going home, until just lately. Now I somehow have the feeling that something is going wrong. I tire more easily and there is a steady and gradual loss in weight. In spite of these symptoms I am trying to convince myself that it's all my imagination. Then Miss Clement came in and said that she is concerned over my weight loss etc. so that only adds to my fears.

November 17, 1942

Dr. Carmichael examined me and said my chest sounds worse and he can now hear moisture on my left side. If the x-ray confirms his suspicions, I will be put back to bed and they will attempt to give me pneumothorax.[6] However, the doctors do not think that I will be able to take pneumo as there are too many adhesions. This is the result of having had pleurisy in 1939.

November 18, 1942 (evening)

As I walked down the street alone this afternoon I experienced some of the darkest moments of my life. I felt certain that there is no mistake and I will be going back to bed. And then a succession of thoughts raced through my mind. How can I tell my parents? They are so sure that I will soon be home. I love the outdoors so much. Now I will be stuck inside again. If only a person could run away from their problems – I would run right out to the West Coast. But when I would arrive there, I would still have TB so I can forget about running away. Does getting drunk really drown a person's problems? If it does, I sure would like to get drunk, just this one time. I am sixteen years old and what plans can I make for the future?

There were no tears shed but how my heart cried as I walked down the street this afternoon. I know that I shall never forget this lonely walk and all those gloomy thoughts that I had today. Even if I am lucky enough to recover and live for many more years these memories will always be a part of me.

---

6 "Pneumothorax is a collection of air or gas in the chest or pleural space that causes part or all of a lung to collapse." http://www.answers.com/topic/pneuomothorax, 29/04/2010. "Lying quietly in the chest like a balloon, the lung has a chance to heal. Later, it may be allowed to inflate again and breathe as before. Sometimes only a part of the lung is collapsed. Collapse of the diseased lung also closes any holes in the lung that may have been caused by the disease. In such cavities, there are thousands of tuberculosis germs and these may be coughed up or spread to other people. In Canada, the first artificial pneumothorax treatment was given in 1898 by a family physician at Ingersoll, Ontario. Patients in Canada would look forward to visiting 'Pneumo' once or twice per week during their stay at the sanatorium." http://www.lung.ca/tb/tbhistory/treatment/pneuo.html, 04/05/2010.

November 24, 1942

Doctor Carmichael put me back to bed. My stomach lavage is negative.[7] My sedimentation is ten. My x-ray has worsened. And I am broken-hearted!

A few days later

Doctor Carmichael attempted to give me pneumothorax but just as was expected, adhesions made it impossible to inject the air into me. Dr. Carmichael and Miss Clement were very sympathetic.

Christmas Day 1942

We were allowed to go home for the day and it was nice being with the family again. Mr. Alex Roger drove me home this morning and brought me back this evening. Everyone is so kind.

February 1943

Things are really going badly. First I started off with a cold and then I began to raise sputum which is positive four.[8] This is my first positive test ever. My x-ray was again worse than the previous one. The doctor and nurses have said that I always obey the rules and yet I keep getting worse. Lord, what next?

---

7   "Lavage is the irrigation or washing out of an organ or cavity, as of the stomach." http://medical-dictionary.thefreedictionary.com/gastric+lavage, 04/05/2010. A stomach lavage could reveal the presence of tubercule bacilli, indicating active disease.

8   "Sputum is the mucus and other matter brought up from the lungs, bronchii and trachea that one may cough up and spit out or swallow. The word "sputum" is borrowed directly from the Latin "to spit." Also called expectoration. "http://www.medterms.com/script/main/art.asp?articlekey5539, 04/05/2010. "Checking the sputum is the best way to find out if you have TB disease." http://www.health.state.mn.us/divs/idepc/diseases/tb/factsheets/sput.., 04/05/2010.

Visits from the clergy help a great deal at these times. Father Latendresse came to visit me for the first time. He is the Parish Priest from Billings Bridge. Then there were Fathers Finn and Gratiana. Father Gratiana sang Italian songs for us and said that anyone with Italian blood should be able to sing. I wonder what happened to me?

April and May 1943

Things are getting progressively worse. Temperature up to 104 and I have pains and pleurisy in my left side again. Doctors say my left side sounds so juicy as the disease continues to spread. I cough a great deal and my sputum is 'positive G six'. Dr. Carmichael told me that I need thoracoplasty surgery and I will have several ribs removed.[9] Nurse said Doctor Carmichael just dreaded having to tell me the bad news and that he feels so sorry for me.

However, there is one great blessing. Doctors say that my right lung is still perfect.

Due to lack of energy I discontinued curling my hair and now wear it in braids. It is so much easier to care for this way.

June 10, 1943

During a severe coughing spell I took a haemorrhage from my lung and that is a frightening experience.[10] I was taken off the balcony and moved into a room alone. Then I was given the usual doses of calcium, and a supply of cracked ice to suck on.

---

9   "Thoracoplasty is the surgical removal of ribs to gain access during surgery or to collapse the chest wall and a diseased lung." http://medical-dictionary. thefreedictionary.com/thoracoplasty, 29/04/2010.

10 An haemorrhage is an expectoration of blood, in this case caused by tuberculosis of the lungs. Usually the haemorrhage comes on suddenly, sometimes after exertion or coughing, while at other times it can come on during sleep.

Next Few Days

Miss Clement is caring for me and it is a comfort having her around. Father Latrendresse came to visit me and said he will return when I am a little stronger and then he will make me a 'Child of Mary'.

I received a letter from Helen Viste in Alberta and she enclosed a gopher's tail to remind me of my childhood in the West. It is so good to have something to chuckle about at this stressful time.

Finally all the haemorrhaging and staining has stopped and I am back on the balcony again with my friends. I was told that from now on I have to be bathed in bed. No more soaking in the bathtub.

July 28th, 1943

There was a lawn party for the patients of the Preventorium and to my surprise Doctor Carmichael allowed me to attend. He said he would be there and everyone would take very good care of me. Dr. Carmichael had his picture taken with the patients and it was a very enjoyable afternoon.

A Few Days Later

Doctor Carmichael left on holidays and Doctor Robert Pritchard took over at the Preventorium. He is a very pleasant young doctor and everyone likes him.

Father Latendresse returned as promised and made me a 'Child of Mary'.

I received a letter from Sister St. Mildred and she is back in Alexandria teaching. She always writes faithfully and still prays for me and for all of her former students.

Last Week of September 1943

The Carmichaels celebrated their 25th wedding anniversary and the patients from all three buildings contributed money to buy them a silver tray. The day after their celebration Doctor Carmichael brought us some lovely cakes and sandwiches that were left over from the party that was held in their honour. Doctor Carmichael also gave each of us girls on the balcony a free raffle ticket.

Month of October 1943

The patients have made a lovely surprise party for me as I am supposed to be transferred to the Whitney Building soon for surgery.

Sunday, November 21st, 1943

Dick Doherty brought Mother, Louis and Billy to visit us and I was so happy to see Billy again. I spoke to Billy through the window as children are not allowed to come inside and he was all smiles as he stood there underneath the window. He has a very nice disposition and I am so proud to be his Godmother.

A friend of Mother's once remarked that she has a feeling that Billy isn't too long for this world. She said he is too happy and pleasant all of the time and for that reason she feels he will die young.

Tuesday, November 23rd, 1943

I was transferred to the Whitney Building and put into Room 15, Third Floor. This is a small room. They want me to be alone as I am going to be operated on tomorrow.

My sputum test is positive G six. My sedimentation is ten and my haemoglobin is 93%.

The Priest came to see me and to hear my confession. There are many people praying for me and I am praying very hard too.

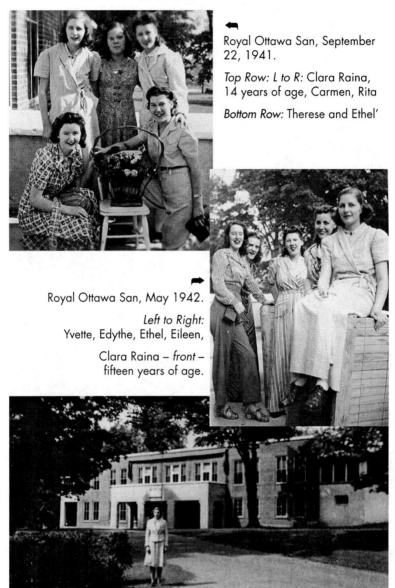

Royal Ottawa San, September 22, 1941.

Top Row: L to R: Clara Raina, 14 years of age, Carmen, Rita

Bottom Row: Therese and Ethel'

Royal Ottawa San, May 1942.

Left to Right:
Yvette, Edythe, Ethel, Eileen,

Clara Raina – *front* –
fifteen years of age.

Clara Raina in front of Preventorium, May 31, 1942, fifteen years of age. The white part of the Pre on the right hand side, with the large windows, was the Balcony.

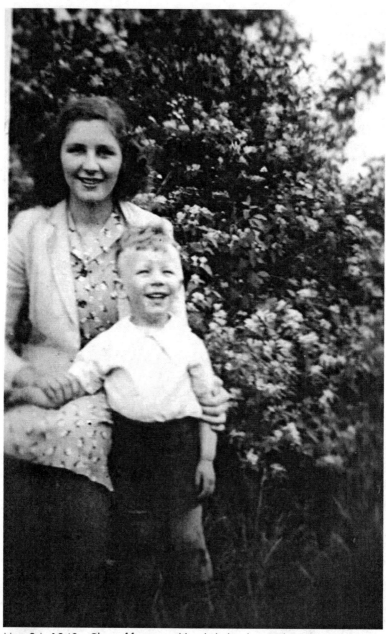

May 24, 1942. Clara, fifteen, and her little brother and Godson, Billy, two years old.

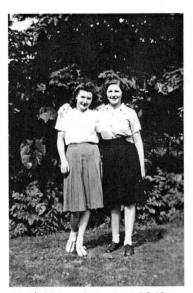

Royal Ottawa San – June 1942.
Clara on right, fifteen years of age,
and Therese.

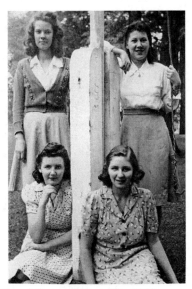

Royal Ottawa San – July 1942.
Standing L to R: Doris and Ethel
Sitting L to R: Therese, Clara Raina,
fifteen years of age.

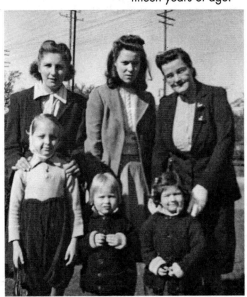

Royal Ottawa San, 1942.
Back Row: L to R. Clara Raina, fifteen years of age, Doris, Ruby.
Front Row: Jeanie, Enid, Connie

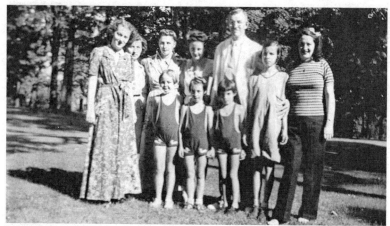

Picnic at Royal Ottawa Sanatorium, July 28, 1943. Dr. Carmichael with the gang of patients.

Back Row: L to R: Corona, Mary Raina, Clara Raina, Rita, Dr. Carmichael, Gladys, Yvette

Front Row: L to R: Connie, Lila, Pearl

The following is a quote of Clara's from the back of this picture.
"Corona, Rita, Yvette and Connie all died of TB. What heartaches."

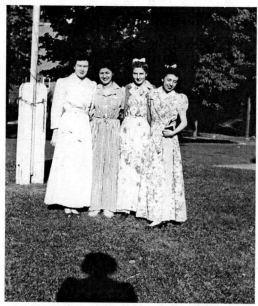

Royal Ottawa San – 1944. *L to R:* Dorothy, Victoria, Clara Raina, Yvette

CHAPTER SEVEN

RIBBED AND DE-RIBBED

November 24, 1943 – December 4, 1944
Seventeen Years, One Month – Eighteen Years, Two Months

Wednesday, November 24ᵗʰ, 1943

When I was wheeled into the operating room I became very curious and wanted to see as much as possible.

However, as soon as I laid eyes on Doctor Lehman in his white cap, I got the giggles and once again it was a time of great embarrassment for me. I would not reveal the cause of my merriment even when Doctor Lehman and the nurses prodded me for an explanation. Well, at least that was until a nurse bent over and whispered this question to me, "Is it Doctor Lehman you are laughing at? He does look so comical." I thought this nurse would be my confidante and I nodded "yes." Then my secret was revealed to all and there was good-natured laughter as Doctor Lehman proceeded to give his opinion on the matter of white hats, etc. He emphasized that I did not look any better than he did, in my garb.

After the laughter had subsided it was time for Doctor Lehman to put me to sleep. Then Doctor Carmichael removed three ribs from my left side with the assistance of Doctor Robert Pritchard.

One of the nurses had told me that Dr. Carmichael usually spoils the patients that he operates on and I soon learned there is a lot of truth in what she said. When it was time to remove my arm from the sling in the evening Dr. Carmichael said that he had already hurt me enough for one day; then he asked Dr. Lehman to do the chore. Dr. Carmichael continued to tell Doctor Lehman that I have always been a good patient and never give them any trouble. Doctor Carmichael made it sound as though I am very special. God Bless these dear doctors!

Mrs. Hodge is on 'Special' with me and she is an excellent nurse. Always pleasant, with a great sense of humour.

December 3rd, 1943

I received some *very* exciting news. Mother gave birth to a daughter in the Grace Hospital in Ottawa and the baby will be named Margaret Anne. Anne is the third daughter and tenth child in our family.

Doctor Carmichael removed the sixteen clips and the stitches from my back – then I was given a clip for a souvenir.

Sunday, December 5th, 1943

Yesterday I had chills and my temperature rose to 101 degrees. Doctor Lehman was on call today and after seeing me he spoke with Doctor Carmichael on the phone. However, Doctor Carmichael still wanted to see me himself so came here instead of going to church and then he wondered if that would be alright with the Lord. He was so worried that he may have given me his cold the other day even though he did not sneeze while in my room.

I am feeling better and everyone here is pleased. Doctors, nurses, my family and clergy are so kind.

Eighteen days after surgery I was allowed out of bed for the first time and my legs were very shaky.

December 20th, 1943

Our beloved Doctor Carmichael is ill and entered hospital for surgery. I am praying hard for his recovery.

Dr. Carmichael's illness will delay my next stage of thoracoplasty. They usually prefer performing these operations three or four weeks apart for best results so the doctor's illness is unfortunate for me as well as for him, only in a much smaller degree.

Christmas Season 1943

The mail is heavy and it is so nice hearing from all of our friends. I received gifts from Ethel and Teresa, the two roommates from 1941 to 1942. We have kept in touch over the years.

Christmas Day, 1943

Dad came to see me and he brought me some pretty little roses.

January 16th, 1944

Mother came to visit for the first time since Anne was born and I was delighted to see her again. I am so eager to meet my new sister but I haven't any idea when that will be.

January 20th, 1944

Happy Day! Doctor Carmichael was in to see me for the first time since his surgery a month ago. He does not look well and we heard that he still has a tube in his stomach.

I am so lonesome for the Preventorium. And for Miss Clement, Miss McDonald and all my other friends but I can't go back until after I have my other operation.

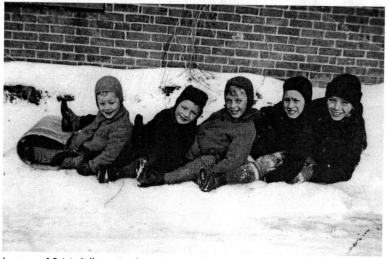

January 1944, Billings Bridge, Ontario.
Left to Right: Billy, Jimmy, Nicky, George and Louis Raina.

February 1944

I read in the newspaper that St. Thomas Aquinas School at Billings Bridge burned down. This was the last school I attended before entering the Sanatorium so the news filled me with sadness as it brought back numerous memories. There was Sister St. Mildred and her everlasting supply of Cod Liver Oil!

Then there was 'Temptation Hill' behind the school that girls were forbidden to slide down. Nevertheless one day I did slide down the hill along with two other girls. As we were climbing back up the hill, Sister St. Mildred was shaking her fist at us and screaming at the top of her lungs. When we reached the top, Sister continued her tirade but then it was directed only at me. "And you, Clara Raina, I always thought that *you* were a young lady. I never thought that <u>you</u> would disobey me – I am so disappointed in *you*." On and on she yelled and my face became redder and redder as more and more pupils congregated to hear what was going on at the top of the hill that winter day.

Dad and Sister St. Mildred were the two most old fashioned people that I knew of at that time but even Dad did not think that it was wrong for girls to slide down a hill.

Now the school is gone and it is time to stop reminiscing.

Last Part of February 1944

My roommate Marcella became very ill so she was moved into a room by herself. Marcella is a lovely girl but she has TB throat so is on 'whisper'. That means she should only speak when necessary and then in a whispering voice.

I have a lively new roommate and her name is Hope.

March 4th, 1944

Dr. Carmichael came in to tell me I should inform my family that I will soon be having my second stage of surgery. Dr. Carmichael brought along a book for me to read.

March 17th, 1944

Marcella died today and she was only nineteen years old. Now her wishes to be buried in a white dress will be granted. Marcella's mother brought the dress to the hospital a few days ago to show her daughter and then they showed it to me.

I used to go in to see Marcella and would pray with her when she was alone. The last visit left me *very* upset. The room felt like death – it seemed *so* cold.

I'll never get used to my friends dying. It is awful.

March 20th, 1944

I will be having my operation the day after tomorrow so things are buzzing. Doctor Carmichael examined me and my Vital Capacity is 75%.[11] My sedimentation is 11 and my haemoglobin is 85%.

Hope will be moved out of this room tomorrow and I will be alone for several days after surgery.

Wednesday, March 22nd, 1944

Dr. Carmichael removed four more ribs from my left side so that makes a total of seven ribs out. Doctor Lehman gave me the anaesthetic and Doctor Pritchard assisted Doctor Carmichael. Doctor McIntosh was also in the operating room but I don't know what part he played.

A Few Days Later – Relating to the Night of Surgery

There was a shortage of 'Special Nurses' and none were available for me until eleven at night when Mrs. Hodge would take over. Thus it was arranged that a practical nurse would assist the regular nurse until 11 p.m. I shall refer to this woman as Mrs. Good because she always gave the patients what they wanted whether or not it was good for them.

The regular night nurse remained with me most of the night except when there was medication to give out and then Mrs. Good took over.

From the moment that I awakened after surgery I kept repeating "May I have a cold drink of water please?" Doctor

---

11 "Vital Capacity is the maximal volume of air forcefully expelled from the lungs after a maximal inspiration. It is a measure of the maximum amount of air the lungs can breathe in or out. A person whose vital capacity is less than 75% of the expected value is generally advised to consult a doctor for further testing before exercising vigorously." http://www.answers.com/topic/vital-capacity, 04/05/2010.

Lehman had jokingly remarked, "Isn't it a shame Clara, but no one is paying any attention to you."

That was until evening when Mrs. Good and I were alone. Then when I asked for a cold drink, Mrs. Good rushed out to get me a large glass of water with ice cubes in it. I hastily drank all the water lest the night nurse return and put a halt to the heavenly treat. As a rule I use common sense but when a person is drifting in and out of consciousness after surgery, they aren't always capable of using proper judgment.

When the nurse took my pulse a few minutes later she hastily sent Mrs. Good to call Doctor Lehman. Then the nurse and Mrs. Good rubbed my legs and the one free arm until the doctor arrived.

No sooner had the doctor entered the room when my stomach turned. Then, in reply to his question, the nurse said that I was still only getting the odd sip of warm water.

"There's a hang of a lot here for just the odd sip of water," roared Doctor Lehman. Mrs. Good remained silent during the entire dialogue.

At this point I felt that death and I were waging a major battle and I feared who the winner might be. My eyes remained closed most of the time and I only saw what was going on when Doctor Lehman would pry open my eyes to examine them with a light. I wanted to ask him if I was going to die but decided against it as I lacked the energy that was needed for speaking. Anyway the doctor would not say "yes," that I was going to die, I concluded. My speech consisted of a grunted "yes" or "no" when questioned by the doctor.

Doctor Lehman was very concerned and he remained with me until my pulse improved and I was feeling better.

The next day the nurse said they had feared that they were going to lose me the previous night. I wondered to what degree the cold drink was responsible for the relapse? I never did tell the doctor as I didn't want to cause trouble for Mrs. Good.

Friday, March 31st, 1944

Doctor Carmichael removed my stitches and then he took down the "No Visitor" sign that had hung outside my door since March 22nd. I have received excellent care from all of the doctors and nurses but my progress has been slow since surgery. Mrs. Belle Powers encourages me to eat. Doctor Pritchard pops in for cheerful little chats. He knows how much I miss the Preventorium and tries to keep me happy – he is very kind. Hope was brought back in so I am no longer alone.

After supper Doctors Carmichael and Pritchard brought in a 'two pound shot bag' that I will have to wear underneath a tight binder to help keep the upper part of the left lung collapsed. The 'shot bag' is made of cloth and it is divided into four sections and each section contains half a pound of BB shots like those that are used in a BB gun.

> (For the next five and a half months the 'shot bag' was removed only twice weekly – just long enough for me to take a bath and then it was replaced underneath a clean binder.)

Monday, May 1st, 1944

Dr. Carmichael came to give me the results of my x-ray. It appears as though my operations have been successful but there is still a wee shadow at the bottom of my left lung. My right lung continues to remain perfect – thank goodness. The sputum tests results are – one test negative – the next one is positive two. That is a disappointment.

I can take tub baths with the nurse assisting me. I still feel very tired and I wonder why.

Our little brother Billy is ill and was in the hospital but the doctor couldn't diagnose his illness so allowed our parents to take him home again.

Saturday, May 13th, 1944

Dr. Carmichael drove me back to the Preventorium in his car and I am so happy to be among my friends again.

The other day I asked Doctor Carmichael if I could go home to see Billy but he said I wasn't well enough to go out.

Sunday, May 14th, 1944

Louis was here and he told me that Billy is back in the Civic Hospital again. He is unconscious. He has meningitis and there is no hope for his recovery. I feel rather numb.

Friday, May 19th, 1944

I was ill when I awoke this morning and my temperature was 102.4. The doctor examined me and took blood tests but they don't know what is wrong.

Ralph came after rest period this afternoon to inform me that Billy died at nine o'clock this morning. Billy, who was only four years old in January. He was a very bright little boy and always so good natured and lovable.

I asked permission to go to Billy's wake but Doctor Carmichael said that with the fever I am running, even walking down the stairs here would be too much for me. Then I would probably cry the whole time and come back much worse than I am now.

Sunday, May 21st, 1944

Billy was buried today and I wasn't able to go to his funeral. After the funeral, Dad and Mother came and they brought wee Anne along with them. The nurses moved my bed close to the window so I could look down and see my little sister for the very first time. She is a little darling and I longed to hold her.

So much joy and such deep sorrow all in the same day.

Sunday, June 11th, 1944

My six year old brother Jimmy came along with Dad this afternoon and I was very happy as we chatted through the window. Jimmy made his First Communion today and he is a fine wee fellow. However, we are very concerned over him as he is having a difficult time getting over Billy's death. There wasn't quite two years difference in their ages and they were very good friends.

Monday, July 3rd, 1944

Dr. Carmichael drove some of the girls over to the Whitney for x-rays and then he took us for a long drive in his car. This was a treat for all of us.

Sunday, July 16th, 1944

Doctor Pritchard gave me the day off and I was overjoyed as it was over eleven months since I had been home. It was so exciting to be able to have a close-up view of my sweet little sister Anne. A wonderful, wonderful day!

Later in July 1944

Things are looking up. Both sputum tests are negative. Sedimentation rate is twelve and haemoglobin is 98%.

Friday, August 18th, 1944

I am tired out! Last week we got two new roommates, Laura and Gwen. Gwen cries most of the time and no matter how hard we try, it is impossible to console her. She is very spoiled and only thinks of herself.

Monday, September 11th, 1944

I am sick and my temperature is over 101. There is a pain in my right side that feels like pleurisy but the doctor examined me and he can't hear anything. My right side has always been perfect but now I am worried. I am still losing weight and that isn't good.

The doctor discontinued the binder and two pound shot bag that I have been wearing since March. He said I might be able to breathe easier without the tight binder across my chest.

Saturday, September 16th, 1944

My temperature is 102 and I still get pains in the right side of my chest. I think that I do have pleurisy. I had pleurisy twice on my left side and I know what pleurisy pains feel like. However, the doctors are very good and they tell me that they can't hear a thing on my right side.

I even asked Miss Clement if the doctors really didn't hear anything, or if they just refrained from telling me as they might think that I would become discouraged if told the truth. Miss Clement assured me that if the doctors heard anything, she wasn't told about it. I am very puzzled!

Sunday, September 17th, 1944

I experienced a very bad night as numerous thoughts raced through my mind. As I tossed and turned I prayed to God that my right side was still alright. Then I came to one conclusion.

I was certain that there was either one of two things wrong with me. I knew there was pleurisy on my right side or else I was suffering from a nervous breakdown for being so sure of having an imaginary illness. I did not like the verdict. If I have pleurisy, my lung will probably become involved. On the other hand, if it isn't pleurisy and I am having a mental breakdown, what will become of me?

Then my thoughts went back to when another patient had a sudden breakdown and all the things she did and the things that she imagined. Will I begin to hear voices telling me to jump out of the window or to throw things at the doctors and nurses? If I really am mentally ill, I hope that they will send me to Brockville before I will injure myself or someone else.[12]

With these thoughts in mind, I fell into a restless sleep but was suddenly awakened with another sharp pain in my chest. Why can't the doctors hear anything! Then I took another deep breath and there was no pain this time. I must be insane, I began to think again. One deep breath brought pain but the next breath brought nothing, so I laid there in total confusion as I prayed and I wept.

More restless sleep. More pains. More prayers and tears, as the night turned into morning.

By the time the day nurses arrived on duty I was very ill and my temperature was 103. Later on Doctor Pritchard examined me and when he put the stethoscope to my chest I knew from the expression on his face that now something could be heard. Then I was told that I have pleurisy with fluid building up. I could tell that Doctor Pritchard and Miss Clement both felt badly and I was shattered.

---

12 Brockville Psychiatric Hospital at Brockville, Ontario, now renamed the Brockville Mental Health Centre.

After Dr. Pritchard was gone I wept for a while and everyone left me alone with my tears. Then Miss Clement returned and told me that I couldn't afford to feel sorry for myself nor to shed any more tears as I would need all of my breath to get better. She is so right, as my breathing is very bad. A large part of the left lung is collapsed as the results of the seven removed ribs. Now with the pleural fluid on the right side, part of the right lung is also out of commission.

Monday, September 18th, 1944

My breathing is bad – I can't eat – and I am very ill.

When Doctor Carmichael examined me today he said that the pleurisy has been working on me for a long time and now they know the reason for my poor appetite and why I never picked up the way that I should have since my last operation.

Doctor Carmichael is very disappointed with this latest change in my condition. Nurse said that he repeated the following phrase to almost everyone that he spoke with. "Poor little Clara, I feel so sorry for her. We just get one side fixed up and now she starts all over again on the other side."

Friday, September 22nd, 1944

Miss Margaret McDonald has returned from her holidays and I am pleased as she is a wonderful nurse and can make a patient feel so comfortable.

I am desperately short of breath and am feeling worse every day. Doctor Pritchard is away on holidays and Doctor Carmichael is keeping a close watch over me.

Miss Burris, the nurse on night duty frequently changes my bed clothes and bathes me as I get wringing wet with perspiration.

The nurses wait on me hand and foot and I'm not even allowed to wash my own face.

I am afraid to fall asleep as I seem to choke and wake up gasping. I would like to try to receive the Last Sacrament but I won't admit that I am that ill as I am so afraid that they will transfer me to the Whitney Building, where they usually place the patients who are dying.[13] For many reasons I sense that they do have the Whitney in mind so I continue to play dumb and refuse to admit how sick I really feel.

There are times that I wonder if the priest would secretly anoint me but then figure that it couldn't be done so am trying to remain in the state of grace and be on the good side of God. However, it would be a great relief to be anointed as I could then peacefully fall asleep without the fear of dying.

Saturday, September 23rd, 1944

My stomach turned, my breathing is bad, I am very ill.

Dr. Carmichael looked so worried while sitting on my bed taking my pulse and respiration. He would like my temperature to subside before aspirating the fluid from my chest.

Monday, September 25th, 1944

This was the day decided upon for aspiration and Doctor Carmichael instructed the nurse to have me arranged lying on my side as I was too ill to be sitting up in the usual position for

---

13 "Last Rites is another term, very common in past centuries but rarely used today, for one of the seven sacraments, the Sacrament of the Anointing of the Sick, which is administered both to the dying and to those who are gravely ill or about to undergo a serious operation, for the recovery of their health and for spiritual strength. The sacrament was called last rites because it was (at least until recent years) usually administered when the person receiving the sacrament was in grave danger of dying. This sacrament is also known as The Sacrament of the Anointing of the Sick, or Extreme Unction." http://catholicism.about.com/od/thesacraments/g/Last_Rites.htm, 23/08/2010.

this treatment. Then Doctor Carmichael removed 300 ccs of pleural fluid before quitting. He said he had to stop because I was passing out on them but that he may aspirate again another time.

Tuesday, October 3rd, 1944

I feel a teeny weeny bit better and my temperature is beginning to go down.

Doctor Carmichael had me listen to the different sounds that could be heard when he snapped his fingers on my chest. Where the sound is loud and clear is where the fluid has cleared up. And where the sound is dull it means that there is still fluid in that area. Doctor Carmichael explained that if I snap my fingers the right way that I will be able to keep track of how much fluid remains on my chest.

More from October 1944

The nurses have been doing everything for me the past few weeks except for making it possible for me to look at myself in the mirror. However, I finally managed to have one of the other patients get the mirror for me.

When I saw my reflection I knew why the nurses had refused to get the mirror. What a shock! How can anyone look this sick and ugly and still be above the ground? My poor roommates! How can they bear looking at this emaciated creature? Now I understand the look of horror on Father Latendresse's face when he came to visit me. Then there were other people who seemed to need a few moments to get their composure after entering the room.

It took me a few days to get over the shock and I was so embarrassed for people to see me like this.

End of October 1944

Miss Evans, our night nurse, is retiring and we honoured her with a farewell party. The celebration took place in this room as I am unable to get out of bed. And since I have been here the longest, I was chosen to read the farewell speech.

Miss Evans has been the regular night nurse at the Preventorium for many years and there are numerous humorous incidents to remember her by so she will not be soon forgotten.

Father Gratton has a newly ordained priest assisting him at St. Bonaventure's Parish and as hospital Chaplain. Father Campeau is fast becoming a great favourite with the patients as he is so understanding to the needs of the sick.

Father Campeau was born on December 29th, 1918 and was raised in Ottawa. He is the son of Adeline Tassé and Albert Campeau, and Father has several brothers and sisters. Father received his education at Saint Charles Parish School, the Ottawa University and at the Diocesan Seminary and there received his Bachelor of Arts Degree in 1940. From there it was on to the Grand Seminary and then Father Campeau was ordained on June 4th, 1944.

Father Latendresse also has a newly ordained priest assisting him at Billings Bridge and his name is Father Leo Lacroix. Father Lacroix came to visit me and he seems to be very nice. He was ordained on June 4th, the same day as Father Campeau was ordained.

Father Montour is another kind priest who often comes to visit the patients and we always look forward to these visits from the clergy.

November 4th, 1944

Today is our parents' Silver Wedding Anniversary. Just wishful thinking, but it would be nice if I was able to join in the little celebration that the family is having at home. Collectively we got our parents a pair of blankets.

End of November 1944

Miss Clement weighed me and I gained four pounds. I am beginning to pick up and am much happier with my reflection when I look in the mirror. However, Doctor Pritchard still says "no" whenever I ask if I can get up for bathroom privileges.

Miss Margaret McDonald quit working here and I miss her and the good care that she always gave me.

Monday, December 4th, 1944

Doctor Pritchard has given me permission to get out of bed once a day to go to the bathroom. I am so excited. I have been a complete bed patient for almost three months this time.

Miss Clement put me on the stretcher and washed my hair for the first time in over three months and it sure felt good.

This has been a very happy day. I had a good shampoo and I was up to the bathroom. My legs nearly collapsed from under me.

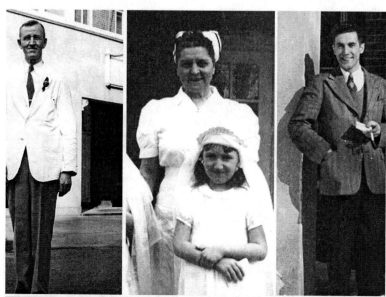

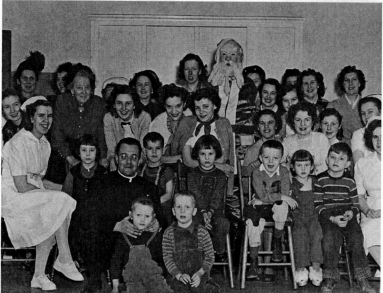

Collage of pictures taken at the Royal Ottawa Sanatorium.
The Three 'Great Cs' and Doctor Pritchard.

Top row L. to R.: Dr. Carmichael, Miss Clement, Jeanie, Dr. Pritchard

Bottom Picture: Father Campeau in the front row.

Clara Raina directly behind Father Campeau.

CHAPTER EIGHT

AVE MARIA

December 1944 – April 15, 1945
Eighteen Years, Two Months – Eighteen Years, Six Months

After Miss McDonald left she was replaced by a nurse who had recently been widowed. I shall refer to this nurse as 'Waxy'.

Mrs. Waxy's late husband spoiled and pampered her and she came to work at the Sanatorium with the hopes that she would also be the centre of attention here. It is a well known fact that her husband was well to do. They were childless and Mrs. Waxy is spreading word around that her will is made, leaving everything to the Royal Ottawa Sanatorium and to some of the patients.

Here in the San the nurses are each assigned a certain number of patients to look after and most of these patients are allowed up for full bathroom privileges. However, Waxy does have one bed patient to look after and I just happen to be that unfortunate creature. Right from the start, Waxy informed me that she did not come here to 'carry bedpans' but came because she is lonesome. Nor does she like to give 'bed baths'. These things make her legs sick. I soon realized that her head is more sick than her legs are!

I am the big thorn in Mrs. Waxy's side and every day she approaches me with a new scheme. Since she just hates carrying bedpans she says "Will I ask to be moved into another room so a different nurse will look after me?" Another plan that she frequently torments me with is, since I have been in the San for years and am really not making any headway, "Why not just quit fighting and allow myself to die?"

Waxy refuses to give up and with every bedpan that she brings and with each bed bath that she gives she lets me know that caring for me is way below her dignity.

To compare Miss McDonald with Waxy is like day and night. Miss McDonald always took very good care of me and never made me feel like a burden. In fact Miss McDonald once said that for my sake she hopes that I will soon be up for bathroom privileges but as far as she is concerned she enjoyed having a bed patient to look after as it makes her feel more like a nurse. I couldn't help but love her and compare her to Waxy. Miss McDonald was always a lady. Waxy is crude and her conversations are usually downright filthy.

Between Christmas and New Year's 1944

Father Campeau gave all of us a pair of prayer beads as a Christmas gift. I think that he is one of the nicest priests that I have ever known.

We had a very pleasant visit from Sister Teresa Ann and she looked lovely in her Religious Habit. Sister Teresa Ann used to visit us as Helen Dunnigan before becoming a nun and we all loved her because of her happy disposition.

Monday, January 1st, 1945

Doctor Pritchard made rounds to wish us all "A Happy New Year." Father Campeau and Father Montour also came to see us and to give their New Year's Blessing.

Mary and Ralph came to see me this afternoon and we had a very pleasant visit. My family never miss visiting day without good cause.

January 12ᵗʰ, 1945

Today Doctor Pritchard gave me the results of my x-ray. There are some spots on the top of my right lung and they are concerned lest these spots might get worse.

Firstly I felt sorry for Dr. Pritchard. He always looks so sad when giving out bad news but he is so wonderfully humane.

Then I felt sorry for myself and uttered a few silent prayers that one of the priests would walk in and be capable of cheering me up. God must have been tuned right in. The prayers were no sooner said when in walked Father Campeau. Father Campeau always seems to know how to handle the sick, and after a few words from him it is easier to smile again.

Middle of February, 1945

Even though I haven't mentioned Waxy for a while, she is still very much with us. We had hoped that by now she would have crawled back into the woodwork but no such luck. She still wants me to quit fighting and allow myself to die. She says she knows other people who had pleurisy and they didn't have to be served with a bedpan. They got up and went to the bathroom. She is so dumb. I hate these old bedpans and would gladly get up, if only the doctors would allow me to.

Waxy did a rotten job of washing my hair on the stretcher and she grumbled the entire time.

A Few Days Later, 1945

Some of the patients asked for my signature on a complaint against Waxy which they had prepared for Miss Stewart, the

Supervisor of Nurses. I refused to sign but told the girls that Waxy has pushed me far enough and I am almost ready to report her to the doctor on my own. One girl promised to eat her undershirt if I actually do report Waxy as I never before have reported on a nurse.

As much as we dislike Waxy we are still able to laugh. Waxy always likes attention and occasionally sings to us, and as she sings she flutters her eyelids and puts on quite a performance. The other day I foolishly remarked that I knew I would crack up if Waxy ever again sings for us. After all the years that I have spent here in the Sanatorium I should have known better than to have made a remark like that.

Later when our supper trays were before us, one of the girls said to Waxy, "Clara just loves your singing, so will you please sing Ave Maria for her?" Waxy was so flattered and hastily prepared for her performance. She came beside my bed and put one of her big fat legs up on the chair, then she opened and closed her eyes as she gave her rendition of 'Ave Maria'. I made every effort to remain calm but my stomach began to quiver and finally the quivering rose up into my throat and I couldn't contain myself any longer. And along with the giggles, up came my whole supper. It was all so unexpected. Consequently I was very thankful for the garbage bag that was pinned to the side of my bed.

Waxy never knew why my stomach was upset but I still chuckle every time that I think about it.

April 6th, 1945

A few weeks ago Father Campeau gave me a little booklet titled, 'The Red Rose of Suffering'. The story is the diary of a TB patient and how she offered one day a week for a missionary priest. She became his co-missionary.

Today Father Campeau and I made a little agreement. He will be the special priest that I will pray for, like a co-missionary. I will offer up one day a week for Father Campeau so he will be successful in his undertakings and for all of his intentions. I hope that I can help Father in some small way like Gertrude did for her priest in 'The Red Rose of Suffering'. Father Campeau will also pray for me.

Friday, April 13th, 1945

Doctor Pritchard put the order in the book that says I can get up and walk to the washroom three times daily. However, I am to continue to have bed baths and to get washed in bed. This still does not satisfy Waxy and she refuses to bring me wash water. When I told Waxy what the doctor had said, she called me lazy and a liar. Our conversation ended when I told her that I will be reporting her to Dr. Pritchard. I know she does not believe that I will actually do it.

Sunday, April 15th, 1945

No sooner had Waxy entered our room when the arguing began. Her tongue was as mean and as filthy as ever. Once again I reminded Waxy that I was going to report her to Dr. Pritchard. Just then Dr. Pritchard entered the room and Waxy made a hasty retreat.

I could see the anger mounting as I was telling Doctor Pritchard that Waxy refused to bring me wash water and accused me of being lazy, saying I just want to be served in bed. Then at this point it was Dr. Pritchard who made the hasty retreat.

A few minutes later a patient from the next room came prancing in and excitedly exclaimed, "You did it Clara, you really did it, you actually reported Waxy to Doctor Pritchard." The patients next door had overheard Dr. Pritchard telling Waxy off and they said that she just kept sputtering and didn't know what to say. This happy girl is the one who is supposed to eat her shirt but we won't hold her to it!

Waxy came in and apologized, which really amazed me. However, she really did get off easy as I never told the doctors or nurses about Waxy suggesting that I allow myself to die.

CHAPTER NINE

THE LITTLE BEAR THAT PRAYED

April 1945 – May 1945
Eighteen Years, Six Months to Eighteen Years, Seven Months

April 1945

Noni made a stuffed toy bear and called it Winganonimous. This toy got a great deal of attention and one afternoon it even received a physical examination from Dr. Pritchard.

We watched attentively as the doctor listened to the bear's chest with his stethoscope and then examined his eyes and ears with a light. Even the bear's reflexes were tested.

Everyone's imagination worked overtime concerning this toy and Noni used a special voice when it was supposed to be the bear that was speaking. We say our rosary beads together every day and that little bear even learned how to pray.[14] And none of us could refrain from laughing when all of a sudden an Our Father or a Hail Mary would be answered in his squeaky little voice.

---

14 "In the Roman Catholic Church, a series of prayers counted on a string of beads. From the Latin word 'Rosarium' meaning 'Rose Garden.' This is an important and traditional devotion of the Roman Catholic Church, combining prayer and meditation in sequence (called decades) of an Our Father, 10 Hail Marys, and a Glory Be to the Father, as well as a number of other prayers such as the Apostle's Creed at the beginning of praying the Rosary." http://www.answers.com/topic/prayer.beads, 04/05/2010.

However, as the saying goes, all good things must come to an end and so it was for us when Winganonimous left the hospital to become a gift for some small child.

Thursday, May 3rd, 1945

Father Campeau is ill and was admitted into the General Hospital. Father Montour suggested we write to Father Campeau and to pray for his recovery. I must pray hard for Father Campeau as he is my special priest to pray for and I sure hope that he is going to be all right.

I have been wearing my hair in braids for two years and it is now seventeen inches long.

Yesterday was a Great Day. The war in Europe ended. We were given the day out today to celebrate V-E Day and I had a very nice time at home with the family. Everyone is happy to know that things are so much brighter war-wise.

CHAPTER TEN

CHICKEN MILK AND
CANNED MALARKEY

May 1945 Continues – December 29, 1945
Eighteen Years, Seven Months – Nineteen Years, Two Months

Month of May 1945 Continues

We were loaded down with goodies from home when we returned to the San on May 8th and among the things that I brought back was a jar of unpasteurized cream. We usually share our treats and when Candy used some of the cream she thought that it was delicious but that it was different from any cream that she had previously tasted. Instead of explaining the difference in the taste was due to the unpasteurization of the cream we told Candy that this white liquid was actually chicken milk.

Candy looked rather doubtful at first and asked many questions. Chickens are so small, how can a person milk them. Why had she never heard of chicken milk until today?

We had an answer for all of Candy's questions. I told her that very few people ever bother to milk their chickens but I have five brothers so things are different with us. Each brother sets a chicken up on a box and then he milks. With five people milking at the same time they are soon able to fill a small jar with the delicious liquid.

During the next few days 'chicken milk' was the topic that was discussed most of the time at our end of the Preventorium. We had forewarned all the other patients to go along with the joke if they were asked any questions on the subject of chickens.

I must admit that Candy did have her moments of doubt and we felt certain that by merely suggesting that she ask Dr. Pritchard she would be convinced. We all knew that Dr. Pritchard could be relied upon to give an honest answer to our questions so when Candy agreed to carry out our recommendation we felt the curtains were about to come down on our lies.

The next time Dr. Pritchard made rounds Candy asked him the all important question. "Do chickens really give milk?" I can still see the look on Dr. Pritchard's face. There was a half smile, a nod of the head, and then he said "Chicken Milk, yes, Chicken Milk – it goes with Canned Malarkey." Then, still smiling, the doctor walked out of the room.

We thought the fun was over but Candy was the first to speak. "What is Canned Malarkey?" she asked.

"Canned Malarkey is a very expensive meat that comes in small tins" one of us replied. "How come I have never heard of Canned Malarkey?" Candy again questioned. "Because this meat can only be purchased where unusual and expensive foods are sold." We knew all the answers.

Doctor Pritchard doesn't know what a great help he was to us. Candy said she wasn't fully convinced about Chicken Milk until Dr. Pritchard mentioned it with Canned Malarkey and then she became a believer.

Besides V-E Day, chickens and malarkey, another very important event occurred this month. Waxy quit working here and we all rejoiced at her departure.

We heard that Waxy had pulled the same trick at other hospitals just like she did here at the Sanatorium. She would inform the staff that her will had been made in favour of that particular institution and then bask in all the attention that was showered upon her. Finally, when her fraud got discovered she just moved on to another hospital with her bag of tricks and filthy talk and started all over again.

I feel sorry for Waxy and still pray for her even though I did not like her.

Latter Part of May 1945

I wrote to Father Campeau in the General Hospital at the suggestion of Father Montour and am overjoyed as I received a reply to my letter. This is the first letter that I have received from my 'special priest'. Father enclosed a wonderful little booklet 'Lift Up Your Hearts'. I still offer Friday of each week for Father and hope that I can be of help in some small way.

Early June 1945

The doctors told me to move around a little more as they are planning to send me home for the summer. However, my x-ray is no better and my right side is causing some concern.

Tuesday, June 28th, 1945

I was discharged for the summer and given instructions what to do while at home. Then Doctor Pritchard said the change in food should do me good and help me to put on a few pounds.

Ralph brought me home and Mother had a room downstairs all prepared for me. I am happy to be home but do wish (oh, so much) that I was well enough to lead a normal life.

As The Days Pass

Since my homecoming coincided with the summer holidays, I often get into card games with my brothers. Then there is little Anne to enjoy and there is much excitement over each new word that she uses.

Father Lacroix has been here to bring Communion and to hear my Confession. The priests are always so good and it helps me to be able to accept this illness more cheerfully.

I always look forward to the mail and like to receive news from my friends back in the Sanatorium so was delighted when I heard from Miss Clement and from Father Campeau.

July 30th, 1945

The Government has started to issue 'Family Allowance' cheques and Mother received her first one today. This cheque was for thirty-three dollars and was for Louis, George, Nick, Jimmy and Anne.

Wednesday, August 15, 1945

This is V-J Day and is a holiday so everyone is celebrating. Ralph took me to see Jean, an old roommate from at the San. I really enjoyed the outing as it was my first time away since I came home from the hospital.

Next Three Weeks

We have had many visitors and it was nice seeing all of these people. Eugenie Henry has been a faithful friend since our school days. Barbara and Marion are very generous with their visits. Dick Doherty is always pleasant when he comes around. He is in the Navy and will be going away. Ralph will miss him a great deal I am sure.

Sister St. Mildred sent me a medal from Ste. Anne de Beaupré and said that now it won't be her fault if I don't get better.

Fathers Latendresse and Lacroix continue to come regularly for Confession and Communion. Many of the patients who have been ill for a long time seem to need the comfort and consolation that the priests give to us during Confession so that is why we go so often and not because we have great sins to confess, generally speaking.

Saturday, September 8th, 1945

Teresa and I were invited to Ethel's place for an afternoon lunch and it was a joyous occasion. We talked and laughed about all the good times that we had together as roommates in the Preventorium in 1941 and 1942.

Teresa looks very well but Ethel has had a relapse so is back on the cure at home. Ethel used to have a very hearty contagious laugh but now she can no longer laugh without coughing. And her eyes have lost their happy sparkle and now display a look of deep inner sadness. Ralph took the three of us for a drive in his little car with the rumble seat before bringing me home this evening.

I have said my beads twice daily for almost six months now.

September 20th, 1945

Dad received a letter from Vincent, his nephew in Italy. This is the first news that he has received in years as we were not allowed to correspond with relatives from that country in wartime. As was expected, the letter gave news of deceased relatives. Among the dead are a brother and three nephews of Dad's.

September 29th, 1945

It is nearly two and a half years since I have chewed gum and I am making this sacrifice with the hopes of obtaining a special favour. The days are rather quiet now that the boys are back in school. However, there is still Anne at home to give us many moments of joy.

The Days Pass

Mrs. Roger and her daughter Elizabeth came to see us and they brought me a lovely white blouse. The Rogers have been very good to me over the years. Barbara Lecuyer continues her cheery and ever-faithful visits.

November 29th, 1945

Ralph sold his rumble seat car for $242.00 as he will be going to Alberta for a while.

December 7th, 1945

I was in for a checkup and Dr. Carmichael said that he will put my name on the list to return to the Sanatorium as soon as there is a bed available.

December 14th, 1945

Dick and Jerry were at our place for supper and then they drove Ralph to the station and waited until he departed by train for Alberta.

December 16th, 1945

My friend Ethel died today and I am sure that Teresa must be feeling as sad as I do. Mary and Louis went to Ethel's wake and they took along a Mass card from me.

Christmas Day 1945

I listened to Midnight Mass on the radio and it gave me a lift. Dick and Margaret Doherty came to see us and we enjoyed and appreciated their visit. We had a fairly nice Christmas but we did miss Ralph.

Saturday, December 29th, 1945

Father Lacroix came for Confession and we enjoyed his visit. Mother served coffee and cake.

This was Dad's last working day at the Post Office as he is being replaced by a returned service man. Many men who held down jobs during the war are being laid off to make room for War Veterans.

CHAPTER ELEVEN

THE LETTER ARRIVES

January 1, 1946 – October 26, 1946
Nineteen Years, Three Months – Twenty Years

January 1ˢᵗ, 1946

In the forenoon we all knelt down and received our Father's blessing. This is a customary ritual in many Catholic homes on New Year's Day.

Friday, January 4ᵗʰ, 1946

A letter from Dr. Carmichael arrived today and there is a bed waiting for me in the Preventorium.

Saturday, January 5ᵗʰ, 1946

Father Latendresse brought Holy Communion and I certainly welcomed the comfort of religion today. Later on this morning Mr. Roger drove me to the Sanatorium and I was accompanied by my Mother. As I walked out the door I wondered if I would ever again be coming home to stay. So many of the girls with whom I was in the San are now dead. However, I tried to think of brighter things and am very thankful for the six wonderful months that I had at home.

Miss Clement admitted me and I am in the second room from the front balcony. I was filled with sadness when Mother left – sad for her and sad for me. We are blessed with the dearest Mother in the world and she suffers even more than we do when we are ill.

Doctor Carmichael came and wished me a Happy New Year. He said they will do all that is in their power to make me well again and I have made up my mind that I will do all that is in my power to get better and I hope that God will supply me with the courage that will be needed.

January continues

It was a delight and a great comfort to see Father Campeau again. He can always make it so much easier for me to accept my illness.

Friday, February 1st, 1946

Dr. Pritchard tried to give me pneumothorax on my right side but once again the aftermath of having had pleurisy prevented me from being able to take it. The right side seems to be following the same course as the left side did, only a few years later.

Doctor Pritchard said the doctors will discuss my case to see if there is anything else that can be done. I am thankful that Doctor Pritchard is still here. He is a good doctor – always seems to convey the message that he will never give up as long as the patient keeps on fighting. I think that is the best incentive that any doctor can give to his patients.

Sunday, February 14th, 1946

My visitors brought me a letter from my twelve year old brother Nick and he wrote "My Godmother sent me two dollars for my birthday so I am sending one dollar to you." Once again,

I am filled with emotions and consider that I am fortunate to be a member of this family.

March 7th, 1946

I gave Father Campeau a dollar to say Mass for Evelyn McCormick as she is very ill and was anointed. I first met Evelyn when I was in the Whitney Building for surgery in 1943-1944 and she was a patient in the next room. Evelyn was teaching school when she became ill and she has many talents but the best of all is her great sense of humour.

Evelyn knew that I was lonesome at the Whitney and she concocted many ways of cheering me. The nurses were called upon on numerous occasions to deliver parcels into my solitary room and the sight of these gifts always delighted me as I knew that Evelyn's good humour was about to emerge one more time.

Friday, March 29th, 1946

I met Dr. Carmichael at the Whitney today when I was over having blood tests this morning and he gave me permission to go up and visit Evelyn.

We were delighted to see each other again and Evelyn was eager to discuss the state of her health. She told me that she hasn't much longer to live and how difficult it was at first to accept the thought of dying. There wasn't anyone that she could speak with about her inner turmoil and she was very upset as she had wanted to speak about her feelings.

Then just when she had reached the peak of her anxieties a strange thing happened. Father Campeau entered her room. As she looked up at Father, she was suddenly engulfed in a feeling of total peace. No longer did she feel the need to discuss her anxieties and she was able to accept the thought of dying.

Evelyn asked if I get a feeling of peace whenever Father enters the room. We both agreed that when it comes to handling the sick and dying, there is no other priest more capable than Father Campeau. I am elated with my 'special priest' and must pray more for him as he has so much work to do.

Evelyn and I had a lovely visit but my heart was heavy as I walked out of her room. I knew that I had spoken with Evelyn for the last time.

During the Month of April, 1946

There is one very unpredictable patient in here so the unexpected occasionally happens. Her boyfriend came to visit her one day but she did not wish to see him so she crawled underneath the bed. He begged her to come out but she ignored his pleas. It was like trying to coax a stubborn dog to come out from under the verandah. The boyfriend was very embarrassed and then he left. We felt very sorry for him but nevertheless it was very comical.

Father Campeau came and informed us that he is being transferred on May 1st. I am shocked and saddened with the news. And I am also frightened. Now what will I do if I am dying and Father won't be here to anoint and comfort me?

The nurses are expressing their regrets concerning the transfer and mentioned their awareness of the state of tranquility that Father evokes in the patients of all religions.

Later on in April we were moved on the front balcony for the summer months and I am in the far left hand corner near Myrtle.

May 1st, 1946

Father Campeau came to say goodbye and I am so sad. He is going to take up duties in Chenéville, Quebec.

"Dear God please watch over Father and help him to succeed in his new undertakings."

May 6th, 1946

I received a box of bath powder and a note from Evelyn's mother. Mrs. McCormick asked me to pray for Evelyn as she is very ill. My roommates joined me and we said 'The Litany for the Dying' and other prayers for Evelyn.

Wednesday, May 8th, 1946

Evelyn died today after being a patient here for several years. Another good friend is gone and it is very difficult. I do hope that she has gone to greater happiness.

Friday, May 10th, 1946

Friday is still my special day to pray for Father Campeau and I say this prayer as often as I think of it. "Jesus please bless and protect Father Campeau, keep him free from sin and help him to succeed in all of his undertakings."

May 1946 Continues

I had various tests and the results are not encouraging. My sputum test is up to positive six from positive two. The doctor said that the only thing that could cure me would be thoracoplasty surgery on my right side but they have decided against it. My resistance is not good enough. They are afraid my TB would go wild and spread all over inside of me if they operated. Then the doctor concluded that I will just have to wait until they get a new drug out for TB – if they ever will!

I guess my case is almost hopeless, unless a miracle happens. At least God is giving me ample time to prepare myself.

June 1st, 1946

Miss Clement wheeled Connie and me out on the open balcony this afternoon. Later our supper trays were brought out and we remained there until seven this evening. We both appreciated this wonderful treat from Miss Clement.

Connie and I have been good friends from way back when Connie entered the Sanatorium at about age seven. At that time I taught Connie how to knit and discovered that she was a very sweet little girl. Also we understand each other as we both seem to go back two steps for every step that goes forward.

Later in June

Both Mother and Miss Clement are in the Civic Hospital and I am very worried and am saying many prayers.

Father Maurice Bilodeau, the priest who replaced Father Campeau came to see us and appears to be very nice. However, he is so thin and looks as though he could use one of our beds.

End of June 1946

Mother and Miss Clement are both out of the hospital. What a relief.

Monday, August 26th, 1946

I finished knitting a red sweater for Anne and will start on a cable stitch sweater for myself out of the same wool. The nurses are trying to discourage me from knitting. They say I look worn out. I do find that knitting tires me and when my sweater is done I'll put away the knitting needles.

September 1946

I embroidered a tablecloth with several roses on it for Mother's birthday on September 9th.

September 25th, 1946

Father Bilodeau brought us Holy Communion this morning. Later on today Father Montour and Father Connelly came to visit and we were pleased to see all of them.

I finished knitting my sweater and it is so warm and comfortable. I like it.

Saturday, October 5th, 1946

Myrtle Jennings was the instigator of a pleasant surprise that I received from my roommates. I was handed an envelope, and inside there was three dollars and a note which said, "Permission has been granted from Dr. Pritchard for you to have the day out tomorrow to celebrate your birthday. The enclosed money is for your taxi fare, and you are to surprise your family and arrive home unannounced."

Sunday, October 6th, 1946

I was greeted by a very surprised family when I arrived home this morning and my twentieth birthday was a memorable day spent with loved ones. Dr. David Roger drove me back here this evening.

After 'lights out' I had difficulty falling asleep because of all the happy thoughts that were going through my mind. There are so many wonderful people in the world - Myrtle and all of my roommates, my good family, and the Rogers who have driven me to and from the Sanatorium many times. Please God, bless all of these good people!

Monday, October 14th, 1946

Today is Thanksgiving and we were given the day off to go home. The weather was beautiful, warm and sunny all day.

Mary, Edna and I went to St. Thomas Aquinas Church after dinner to make a visit of thanksgiving. When we emerged from the church the weather was so inviting that we decided to proceed on to the Mayfair Theatre and see a movie. *Road to Utopia* was playing and we enjoyed the show. Another wonderful day.

Mother was frantic when we arrived home as she feared that an accident had befallen us. Our intentions were to only go to church and the store when we left home. We didn't have a telephone so there was no way of notifying the family about our change of plans.

Over the years I have often felt a sense of guilt and remorse for the worry that I caused my dear Mother that day.

Saturday, October 26th, 1946

Dr. Pritchard gave me the results of the tomagraph x-rays that were taken yesterday. There is a cavity about the size of a fifty-cent piece in my right lung. Doctor Pritchard is going to speak with Dr. Douglas Hermann, the surgeon, to inquire if it will be possible to do anything for me, surgically speaking.

I am in a bad situation and need a miracle, I think.

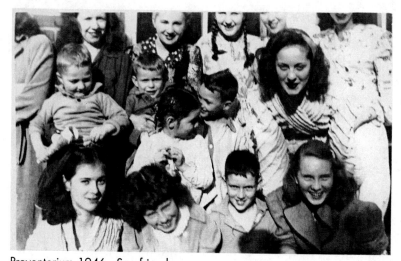

Preventorium 1946. San friends.
Back Row: L. to R. Jeanine, Myrtle Jennings, Clara Raina next to her (with braids), Loretta, Teresa

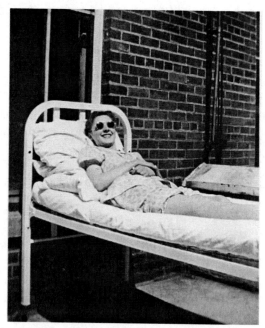

June 1946. Clara in the San, nineteen years of age.

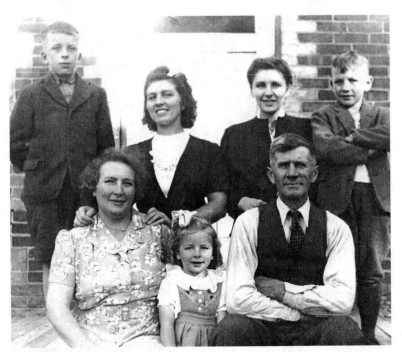

Summer 1946, Billings Bridge, Ontario.
Front Row: L. to R. Mom (Elizabeth Raina), Anne, Dad (Dominic Raina).
Back Row: L. to R. Nick, Mary, Clara, Jim Raina

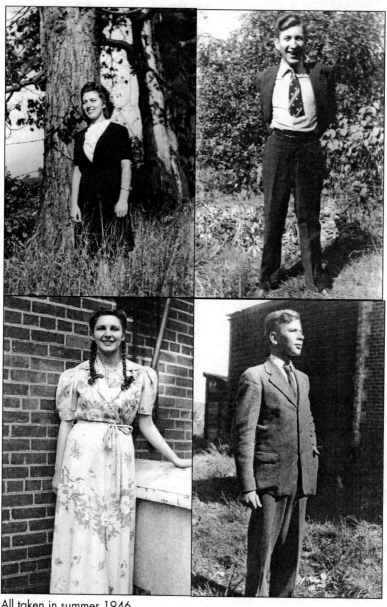

All taken in summer 1946.

Top Row: L to R.   Mary Raina, twenty-three years of age; Ralph Raina,
twenty- one years of age.

Bottom Row: L to R. Clara Raina, nineteen years of age; Louis Raina,
sixteen years of age;

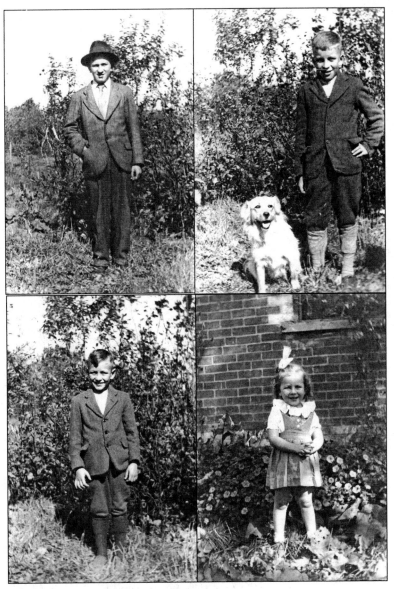

All taken summer 1946.

Top Row: L to R.   George Raina, fourteen years of age; Nick Raina, twelve years of age.

Bottom Row: L to R. James (Jimmy) Raina, eight years of age; Anne, two and one half years of age.

CHAPTER TWELVE

A DIFFICULT DECISION

November 17, 1946 – June 6, 1947
Twenty years, One Month – Twenty Years, Eight Months

Sunday, November 17th, 1946

Doctor Pritchard came during rest period and said that I must be anxious to hear what they have decided to do about me.

Doctor Hermann has agreed to take the risk of performing a thoracoplasty operation on my right side if I am willing to take the risk of having it done. However, Dr. Hermann does not intend to remove more than four ribs (for reasons of breathing) and I may end up being worse off with the surgery but it is my only chance of ever getting better.

I want to risk the surgery and Dr. Pritchard said that he had surmised that I would want it this way.

Friday, November 22nd, 1946

The Cod Liver Oil season opened today and will last until late in the spring. I hate the oil as it tends to repeat on me. Swallowing it once a day is bad enough, but when it keeps repeating, it's like taking it several times daily, similar to the way Sister St. Mildred used to have me do in school.

I was dreading the thought of the long season that lay ahead when the nurse came in and informed me that Dr. Pritchard has ordered vitamin pills instead of cod liver oil for Connie and me. The doctor feels that the oil is too hard for us to digest after all the years that we have been in bed. The other patients must take the cod liver oil. Neither Connie nor I had complained, so Dr. Pritchard is our hero today and will be for the remainder of the winter as we look on while the other patients are swallowing their smelly cod liver oil.

Friday, December 13th, 1946

The Sanatorium in Haileybury is faced with an emergency. They need a doctor to replace the one who has taken ill so Dr. Pritchard will be going there to help them out. We are very sorry and hope the crisis will be of a short duration.

January 1947

In November Dr. Carmichael said that I will have the surgery before Christmas. Then it was going to be right after Christmas. Now he says maybe not until May or June. This last postponement has really upset me as I now feel that Dr. Carmichael is just trying to back out completely.

One thing is certain, without surgery and with a cavity the size of a fifty-cent piece in my lung, my next move will be to the cemetery. And I'm not ready yet to die without a fight. No matter how small my chance is with surgery, I still want this chance.

I have always thought the world of Dr. Carmichael and now I get a little angry and lippy towards him for stalling with the surgery. Then after the lights are out at night, I usually have a little cry because I know that I have hurt his feelings.

I miss Dr. Pritchard. He would fight for me as he is the one who asked Dr. Hermann about surgery in the first place. There are so many people praying for me that 'just maybe' I might surprise everyone and get better if I do have surgery.

January 29th, 1947

Father Campeau was in Ottawa and he came to see me. This really helped to cheer me up. I still pray a lot for Father Campeau and offer one day a week for all of his undertakings. However, I have been so ill-tempered and blue lately, so doubt that my prayers are worth very much.

Dr. Carmichael mentioned that my last x-ray is slightly worse and spoke of surgery again.

Saturday, February 1st, 1947

Dr. Pritchard returned to get his car and his belongings as he is not coming back to the Royal Ottawa Sanatorium. He came to say goodbye and after he left there weren't too many dry eyes around here. We will miss 'Our Doctor Pritchard' and his many words of wisdom. A sad day!

Friday, February 7th, 1947

I made a Holy Hour (one hour of praying) for Father Campeau and all of his intentions. Father Montour was here and he asked me if I would teach two of the younger girls their Act of Contrition as they had forgotten how to say it. The task was easy as both girls learned quickly.

Monday, March 10th, 1947

Dr. Carmichael examined me and is quite certain that I will be having my thoracoplasty operation this Thursday. He said that it is a great risk and if he was still the surgeon that he would not operate on me. He personally thinks that I would live longer without the surgery. The only reason they are going to operate is because I haven't a chance at all without it.

I am a little nervous but I want this operation as it may be successful. I hope the family won't worry nor feel too badly if I don't pull through. I know God will do what is best for me.

My Vital Capacity is 55%.

Tuesday, March 11th, 1947

Dr. Carmichael came after supper and he sat down on my bed, then told me that he cannot allow the surgery to take place. The risk is just too great. The operation is cancelled!

I couldn't utter one word so just turned my head and cried. This is the first time in my life that I have cried in the presence of a doctor. As I lay there crying, Dr. Carmichael said that he will speak with Dr. Hermann again and see if they can come up with anything else. I know he felt badly, but the tears were beyond my control.

Now I realize why Dr. Carmichael kept putting me off about the surgery. He was worried. And I would get so angry towards him. I guess that it isn't always easy being a doctor and most of us would probably do the same if we were in their place.

Wednesday, March 12th, 1947

Dr. Carmichael came in rest period and wanted to know if I am still angry at him. I tried to assure him that I am not angry at him, but am very disappointed as I had wanted this one chance to get better.

Thursday, March 13th, 1947

Doctor Carmichael said he went over my whole case with Dr. Hermann. Since I want the surgery so badly, Dr. Hermann will do a small thoracoplasty operation on me next week.

Dr. Carmichael said that he is now convinced that I will end up hating him if he does not allow the surgery to take place. Once again I tried to reassure the doctor and said that I would never hate him but he thinks that I would. Normally Dr. Carmichael and I get along very well and are good friends. Doctor Carmichael often says that he feels as though I belong to them as they have practically raised me.

Tuesday, March 18th, 1947

Father Gratton came and I went to Confession and received Holy Communion. Miss Clement took up a collection from the nurses and patients of the Preventorium. Then the money was given to me to help to pay for the special nurses that I will need after surgery. There are so many wonderful people in the world. Please God, help me to keep my courage.

Wednesday, March 19th, 1947

I was transferred into a single room in the Whitney Building – Room 12, 2nd Floor. Father Campeau was not aware that I was scheduled for surgery tomorrow but he was in Ottawa and came to see me. God is so good. I think He knows of my great need to receive encouragement from Father Campeau. After Father's visit and receiving his blessing, I am no longer afraid of tomorrow. Dad and Mother came to visit this evening and I wish they weren't so worried over me.

I know how upset Dr. Carmichael is concerning the surgery so I wrote a letter for him and hid it among my belongings. He is only to receive it if I should die. The letter states that I do not want Dr. Carmichael nor anyone else blaming themselves in any way for my death. I am well aware of the risk that I am taking and, if I die now, it only means a little sooner than what was bound to be certain death without surgery.

I want to thank everyone for all the kindness shown to me during the many years of my illness. And I want to wish them all the very best of everything in their future. My family, the staff here at the Sanatorium, the clergy and my many friends have all brought so much happiness into my life during all these years.

Thanks again to everyone. Thus ends the hidden letter.

Thursday, March 20th, 1947

Father Gratton brought Communion and I am well prepared. I can offer my pains for so many things, especially for Father Campeau's work. I put a Sacred Heart Badge in my sock as I prepared to go down for surgery.

I was pleased when Dr. Carmichael popped into the operating room to say "Hi" before I was put to sleep. He said that he knows I am going to be alright because I am still able to smile. Then before Dr. Lehman gave me the anaesthetic I asked "Will you please say a wee prayer for me?" "I sure will" Dr. Lehman replied.

Dr. Hermann removed two ribs and I came through the surgery far better than was anticipated and everyone was elated. Dr. Carmichael had kept a vigil outside the operating room during the entire operation. When I came out he was like an excited little boy and rushed right over to the Preventorium to tell everyone there that I had survived the surgery and all is well so far.

As I marvelled at how well I felt Dr. Lehman cautioned, "Hush, Clara, you are scaring me. Wait until a couple of days have passed before you say how well you feel." I was dozing off and on after surgery when Father Gratton came in to give me his blessing. And I insisted that I had to use my right arm and tried to free it from the sling, despite the fact that Father told me that I could use my left hand to make the sign of the cross. Apparently Father was quite amused with our conversation and later related the details to others. But I have absolutely no recollection of the visit. And I even said to the nurse, "No, the priest has not been in to see me" when she made inquiries about a visit with him.

Saturday, March 22nd, 1947

Dr. Lehman was in at 9:00 a.m. to change my dressing and remove the oxygen tube from my nose, and everyone was still elated with my condition. I remarked that I was very comfortable but felt as though I could sleep for hours when they were through with me. I must have fallen asleep immediately. And the next thing I knew was when the nurse awakened me to use the bedpan around 11 a.m.

I then remarked that I was very sick. My head felt as big as a washtub and my temperature was at least 103. Nurse reminded me that my temperature was near normal at 9:00 a.m. but nevertheless she took it again. I was right. My temperature was way up. Then things began to happen.

Dr. Lehman rushed in and connected me to the oxygen tank. And he was followed by Dr. Carmichael. Doctor Hermann was sent for and he joined the other doctors in my room.

In the meantime there was activity back at the Preventorium. My old roommates and friends had seen Dr. Hermann driving in a bit faster than usual and they rushed up to the desk to ask if I was the reason for the doctor's hasty trip. Miss Clement phoned to the Whitney for information. Then she rushed to each room asking, "Pray harder than you have ever prayed before. Clara has just taken a very bad turn."

Back to the Whitney again. After the doctors left my room the nurse gave me an injection in my hip and that was the first time that I had ever received a needle in that area. I had been given a hypo in my arm a few minutes earlier so I asked the nurse what this needle was for. With a look of doom on her face, she replied "I can't tell you what the injection is for. You are very ill and need plenty of rest so go to sleep. The priest will be coming to see you."

This nurse meant well but her asinine reply made my imagination work overtime. I thought about other times when dying patients had received hypos and the nurses would tell us that they weren't expected to come out of it. Maybe the needle I received was an extra big dose so I wouldn't be aware of dying? Maybe I have TB meningitis? My head does feel as big as a washtub. After all, the doctors were very pessimistic about my chances of recovery and said that surgery might cause my TB to go wild and spread to other parts of my body.

Then I made up my mind. I will not go to sleep, no matter how tired I get. As long as I am awake, I can fight off death. As I lay awake with these thoughts in mind, the three doctors returned from their dinner. "Did you receive your shot of Penicillin yet?" inquired Dr. Lehman. "You will be getting a shot every three hours for a few days." I was momentarily angered and opened my mouth to speak. But hastily got my emotions under control and pursed my lips in silence. My request would have been directed to Dr. Lehman exclaiming "Will you please go grab Mrs. Hypo and give her a swift kick in the backside for me?"

So few patients here at the San have received Penicillin, that it never dawned on me that I had been given this wonderful drug. I had heard that Penicillin once saved Dr. Carmichael's life. If only I had known what I had been given I would have relaxed and allowed myself to go to sleep. I was so desperately tired. If I live to be a hundred I will never forget the horrors surrounding my first shot of Penicillin.

Father Bilodeau did come to give me his blessing. And Miss Clement came to see me. Everyone is kind. Even Mrs. Hypo meant well, but she chose the wrong profession when she went into nursing.

Monday, March 24th, 1947

The three doctors came in together again. And Dr. Carmichael told the other doctors and me about the children in the Preventorium. When he made rounds he heard all this mumble jumble going on among the children of various religions and he asked them what they were doing. "We are praying for Clara" the children replied in unison.

Miss Pearl Walker, the assistant supervisor of nurses, sent me a lovely tulip plant. I am truly moved by everyone's kindness.

Tuesday, March 25th, 1947

Transfusions have to be replaced or there is a fee of twenty-five dollars for each transfusion received. Thus it was that Ralph and Dick Doherty came to see me this afternoon as Dick had been in to replace a transfusion for me.

Friday, March 28th, 1947

Dr. Carmichael told me that I will be having my second operation next week and this news came as a big surprise as it will only be fourteen days between operations and they usually wait three or four weeks.

Wednesday, April 2nd, 1947

I received a lovely little note from Father Campeau and it brought joy into my heart. Doctor Carmichael did various tests in preparation for my surgery tomorrow.

Holy Thursday, April 3rd, 1947

The priest brought me Holy Communion which was a great comfort on this all-important day once more. About a half hour before going down for surgery Miss Cox informed me that Dr. Lehman was ill and arrangements had been made for another doctor to come and give the anaesthetic. I was crestfallen. "Are you saying that you would feel better if grumpy old Dr. Lehman was here?" I assured Miss Cox that I would indeed feel better with Dr. Lehman around. I don't know what transpired after that but before long Dr. Lehman walked into my room. I was jubilant!

And once again Dr. Carmichael popped into the operating room and had a few words with me before surgery. And I asked him if they would save one of my removed ribs for me as I was curious to see what they look like.

Then Dr. Lehman's entry into the operating room brought exclamations of surprise from the medical staff. And again he said that he wonders who would start the rumour that he was ill. A strange doctor was there to administer the anaesthetic and Dr. Lehman sat on a stool by my head. My last thoughts were "How nice of you Dr. Lehman, but you aren't fooling me. By the way you look, you will be out of here as soon as I am asleep." My surmising was entirely erroneous. In spite of being so ill, Dr. Lehman remained on the stool and kept his eyes on me until the surgery was completed. So often we tend to complain about the medical profession and forget to mention the occasions when they give so freely of their time and service, even when they may be very tired or are quite ill themselves.

Doctor Hermann removed two more ribs which makes a total of four out of my right side. My condition was considerably worse during and after surgery today than what it was two weeks ago.

Dr. Lehman's intentions were to give me a blood transfusion but his many attempts were in vain instead of in vein. Finally he moved down to my ankle and removed my sock. Inside he found the Sacred Heart Badge that I had smuggled down to surgery. He handed the Badge to the nurse and asked her to pin it on my gown. Then followed several more failures to set up the transfusion. Finally Dr. Lehman put down the equipment. He took a deep breath and then my ears heard for the very first time all those curse words that had earned Dr. Lehman a reputation of his own. The sudden shock of hearing these words must have caused my adrenalin to flow which in turn improved my blood circulation because the next needle went in like a charm. Then Dr. Lehman looked down at me and said "You know Clara, cussing really does help and you should try it the next time that things are going wrong."

Good Friday, April 4th, 1947

I am not feeling too well and I offered my day for Father Campeau's undertakings. Dr. Hermann was in to see me. Everyone is very kind.

Saturday, April 5th, 1947

Another difficult day. Stomach very upset. Dr. Lehman changed my dressing and wanted to know what was worrying me. I tried to assure him that I was extremely tired, not worried. I received a cheerful Easter card from Dr. Pritchard and was delighted to hear from him.

Dr. Carmichael changed me over to a new tank of oxygen at about 5 p.m. and said that he will be able to sleep much better tonight just knowing that I won't run out of oxygen. When Dr. Carmichael first entered my room with the large wrench in his hand I wondered just how that wrench would be medically used. I soon learned that some oxygen tanks need a good wrench and a strong arm to be turned on.

Doctor Lehman phoned Mrs. Hodge (my special nurse) this evening and asked her to find out what was troubling me. I once again stated that I wasn't worrying, but was extremely tired. Finally Mrs. Hodge left the room, only to return moments later with the empty oxygen cart and then she explained. "Everyone has been telling you that you can expect to be very short of breath as the results of your surgery so I thought that you might be interested in seeing what you will look like when you are walking down the street pushing along your oxygen tank." With that, Mrs. Hodge kicked up her heels and pranced around the room pushing the oxygen cart ahead of her. I laughed so hard and continued to laugh the rest of the evening every time that I looked at Mrs. Hodge.

Later on Dr. Lehman once again phoned Mrs. Hodge and this time he was relieved to hear that I was laughing, even though he was not told the reason for the merriment. I asked Mrs. Hodge why Dr. Lehman was so concerned and why he was so sure that I was worrying. She then quoted Dr. Lehman "Clara hasn't been smiling and when Clara doesn't smile there is something seriously wrong with her." Mrs. Hodge said she believed me when I said that I wasn't worrying but decided that what I really needed was a good laugh. She thought I would see the humour in the oxygen cart escapade. That was very wise judgment on her part as the bout of extreme fatigue gradually disappeared when the laughter had subsided. And I felt so much better. I wholeheartedly agree with the phrase 'Laughter is the Best Medicine'.

Easter Monday, April 7th, 1947

Doctors Hermann, Carmichael and Lehman came in together and were in a good mood. Dr. Carmichael expressed his hopes that I will be alright now as he has not had peace of mind for the last six months as he has worried so much over me. Father Latendresse came this afternoon and he stayed for a long pleasant visit.

Tuesday, April 8th, 1947

Miss Margaret McDonald sent me a lovely bouquet of tulips. Ralph, Mary and Miss Clement were here to see me. This all helps so much as it gets very lonesome when one is in a room all alone.

Wednesday, April 9th, 1947

This was a big day. The nurse brought the rib that I had asked Dr. Carmichael to save for me. It was wrapped in a large wad of paper towelling and was on my bedside table for several hours before I had the courage to look at it. I asked the nurse if she would show it to me but she said that I would have to unwrap it myself. The removed portion of rib is five inches long. And it didn't bother me when I looked at it. Now I will put it away as a keepsake. Dr. Carmichael said they cleaned up my other rib and will use it at a Medical Convention.

Monday, April 14th, 1947

I gave Father Gratton money to say a Mass of Thanksgiving because I survived the surgery. I am so thankful to be alive.

Thursday, April 24th, 1947

Doctor Lehman came when I had the bedpan and he called it my gondola. The doctors often say that I am pale but I know that wasn't the case today.

Saturday, April 26th, 1947

We have to buy our own thermometers and keep them on our bedside tables and consequently they rarely last more than a year before they are broken. My last thermometer was nearly five years old and was becoming a conversation piece. This morning Miss Cox wheeled me out to the balcony on the stretcher so I could visit with the other patients while she changed my bed. All of a sudden she came rushing out to inquire how long I had my thermometer. "For nearly five years" I replied. "That's what I thought you said, but you haven't got it anymore as I just broke it" exclaimed Miss Cox. We couldn't help but chuckle a bit as she did look very comical when she made her confession. However, I did miss my thermometer. We had shared so many ups and downs together!

Monday, April 28th, 1947

Happy, Happy Day! I returned to the Preventorium building today and am in the same room and place as I was before I went to the Whitney. And I am also with the same three roommates, as before; Betty, Aline and Georgette. I can walk to the bathroom once a day but must remain in bed the rest of the time.

End of April, 1947

My three sputum tests are negative under direct smear and that is great news so far. I lost over seven pounds while at the Whitney and now weigh 113 pounds.

Month of May, 1947

Dr. Pritchard was in Ottawa and came to visit us. Everyone was so excited and happy to see him again. Father Campeau came and brought me a box of chocolates. As usual Father's visit left me in a cheerful mood. Miss Margaret McDonald sent me a box of chocolates and a lovely card. People are so good to me.

Sunday, June 1st, 1947

Mother brought Jimmy and Anne along with her and I was allowed to speak to them through the window. Needless to say, I was excited. I had not seen them since Christmas.

Friday, June 6th, 1947

I made a Holy Hour for Father Campeau's intentions. Another wonderful day. Father Campeau came to visit us.

CHAPTER THIRTEEN

THE MARIAN CONGRESS

June 17, 1947 – July 25, 1947
Twenty Years, Eight Months - Twenty Years, Nine Months

Tuesday, June 17th, 1947

Fathers Montour and Latendresse took most of the girls to the Marian Congress in their cars this afternoon.[15] Father Latendresse said he has Dr. Carmichael's permission to take Connie and me to the Marian Congress tomorrow at 9:00 a.m. and we will be going by ambulance. I am very happy as I never thought that I would be able to go so now I can look forward to tomorrow with excitement.

Wednesday, June 18th, 1947

Through the volunteer service of Mr. Racine and his ambulance, Fathers Latendresse and Brisbois, Connie and I were taken to the Marian Congress being held at Lansdowne Park in Ottawa.

The two priests wheeled me into the Chapel on the stretcher to touch the statue of Our Lady of the Cape. At the foot of the statue I met Sister St. Margaret Mary who had taught my younger brothers at St. Thomas Aquinas School at Billings

---

15 The Marian Congress was a large celebration to mark the centennial of the founding of the Archdiocese of Ottawa.

Bridge. I think everyone loves this nun with her warm friendly smile and it was a real joy seeing her today.

The priests took me inside two other buildings to view the Religious exhibits. We spoke with many priests and nuns who promised that they would pray for me and I even received the blessings from a Bishop. Some priests from the States asked if they could take my picture and said that it will be published in the Miraculous Medal Magazine.[16] Mr. Racine carried Connie around in his arms and Miss Currie (a nurse) came along to keep an eye on both of us.[17] Connie and I both agree that there are great people in this wonderful world of ours.

Friday, June 27th, 1947

Father Maurice Bilodeau came to say goodbye as he is being transferred to Hawkesbury. We are sorry to see Father leave as he has always been kind to us.

Lucienne, a patient here at the Preventorium, has started to take the new drug 'Streptomycin'.[18] She had her first injection yesterday. Now we are all hoping, praying and waiting to see if this drug will be our answer for a cure for tuberculosis.

---

16 A few weeks later I received some pictures that were taken at the Marian Congress by the priests of the Miraculous Medal. They also sent me a few copies of the magazine with my picture in it.

17 Miss Grace Currie, the nurse who came along with us, was murdered on February 9th, 1954.

18 "The dawning of a new day occurred in 1944 with Wakeman's discovery of streptomycin, the first specific antibiotic that proved lethal to the mycobacterium (the bacteria causing tuberculosis). Isoniazid and PSA (Para-amino-salicylic acid) quickly followed and their prompt adoption for treatment and the prevention of recurrences produced miraculous consequences. In 1948, some 7.2% of patients received streptomycin. By 1953, 77% of patients were on streptomycin. Para-amino-salicylic acid (PAS) came into use in 1950 and was common by 1952." An History of the Fight Against Tuberculosis in Canada – http://www.lung.ca/tb/tbhistory/timeline/antibiotics.html, 07/05/2010.

'Streptomycin' is the word that is most often spoken around the Sanatorium these days.

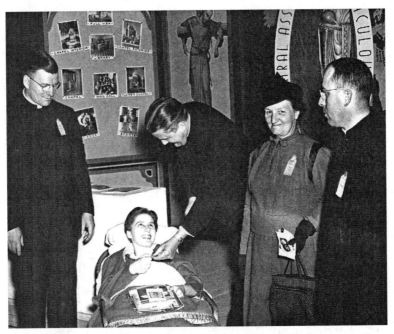

June 18, 1947. The Marian Congress at Lansdowne Park.
Father Latendresse standing to the left of Clara Raina on the stretcher, Miss Currie, Nurse, standing.

Friday, July 25th, 1947

Mother and Dad came to see me and then they went to see Dr. Carmichael. The doctor told my parents that I will be an invalid for life. Otherwise he is satisfied with my condition.

CHAPTER FOURTEEN

THE RAINA FAMILY MOVES TO KEMPTVILLE

July 31, 1947 – September, 1947
Twenty Years, Nine Months – Twenty Years, Eleven Months

Thursday, July 31ˢᵗ, 1947

My parents purchased a hundred and fifty acre farm at R.R. No. 2, Kemptville, Ontario and the family moved there today.

I am filled with emotions over their move as this farm is over thirty miles south from Ottawa. This will mean changes for all of us. I used to have visitors every Sunday when the family lived at Billings Bridge but now they won't be able to come as often to see me. It will also mean a big change when I leave the San to go home as I don't know anyone in Kemptville.

Monday, August 4ᵗʰ, 1947

Doctor Carmichael examined me and things seem to be going well but he can hear râles on both sides of my chest.[19]

---

19 "Crackles, crepitations or râles are the clicking, rattling or crackling noises that may be made by one or both lungs of a human with a respiratory disease during inhalation. They are often heard only with a stethoscope." http://en.wikipedia.org/wiki/Rales, 05/05//2010.

Wednesday, August 6th, 1947

Some men were installing lovely white Venetian blinds on our windows and, while working, they accidentally knocked down my plaque of St. Gemma and broke it. I feel badly as that plaque was given to me by Father Campeau.

The broken plaque was just the beginning of a bad day. Doctor Carmichael told me that my sputum test is positive. The tests had all been negative since shortly after my last operation so this is a real blow. I am so disappointed and so is Doctor Carmichael.

August Continues

There was a lawn picnic for the patients of the Preventorium and Dr. Carmichael allowed me to go for one hour. It was a treat getting outside and I enjoyed the change. Dr. Carmichael is still trying to cheer me up. I think he feels just as sorry for me as I do for myself over that positive sputum test.

René Poulin drove me to the Whitney for the Sterio-x-rays and blood tests. The sedimentation rate is six and my haemoglobin is 90%. We haven't got an elevator in the Preventorium and I was short of breath coming back upstairs.

First Week in September 1947

I received three days leave and this gave me an opportunity to explore our home in Kemptville. The holidays passed too quickly but I did have a lovely time with the family and enjoyed Mother's cooking. Now I can vision what our house looks like when I daydream of home.

CHAPTER FIFTEEN

I WONDER WHO HE IS?

September 22, 1947 - December 31, 1947
Twenty Years, Eleven Months – Twenty-One Years, Two
Months

Monday, September 22ⁿᵈ, 1947

"He looks so kind! I wonder who he is?" My bed is by the window so I have been able to watch the Whitney patients coming outside for lawn privileges all summer.

There is one particular man who I watch for every day. He is the first patient who I have ever been interested in. He looks like a very nice man. And I feel certain that he is a very kind and trustworthy person. I kept this crush a secret until today. Then I just had to ask someone about this man.

I was told that his name is Harold Mouré. He is single. He is very religious but not stuffy. He has a good sense of humour and is liked by everyone. Harold speaks to the girls but has not shown any romantic inclination towards any of them.

This last statement caused my roommates to chuckle. Then they told our informer that I had never shown any interest in men until now. Thus they all agreed that it might be very interesting if the two of us could be brought together.

I would love to meet Harold and can only hope that some day the opportunity will present itself.

Wednesday, September 24th, 1947

Lucienne trimmed a bit off my hair and then she put it up in curlers. I am anxious to see what I will look like with my hair curled as I have been wearing it in braids for four and a half years. It is still long enough to braid so I will probably continue to wear it that way most of the time.

Sunday, September 28th, 1947

The cold weather was the main topic of conversation when Ralph, George and Dick Doherty were here this afternoon. There were also many other visitors in the room when Dick suddenly and loudly exclaimed "Clara is going to knit me a pair of woollen underwear to keep me warm this winter." I blush very easily and turned many shades of red as everyone chuckled at Dick's announcement.

Later this evening I decided that Dick is going to receive a pair of knitted long johns. Then I got out some red and green wool and knit a miniature pair of underwear, trapdoor and all.

Monday, September 29th, 1947

Dr. Lehman made rounds and Mrs. Boles showed him the little pair of underwear that I knit. They are receiving a great deal of attention so I will wait until the excitement has died down before I mail them on to Dick.

Monday, October 6th, 1947

I am twenty-one years old today and I received several lovely cards and presents. Lucienne made me a swan out of sea shells and she wrote 'Harold' on it. I hope the day will come when I can actually meet this gentleman.

There is a big beautiful tree outside my window and now the leaves are in the process of changing colours. This tree is also very popular among the black squirrel population. And on numerous occasions we can see several of them scurrying among the branches all at the same time. During the long periods I am confined to bed I like to look at the trees.

Saturday, October 18th, 1947

The day was bright and beautiful and the leaves are gorgeous so when Dr. Carmichael made rounds I asked for a very special favour. I requested his permission, just for today, to go outside and sit on the bench underneath the tree by my window. Dr. Carmichael granted me my wish and I was elated.

No sooner was I seated on the bench this afternoon when the other patients swung into action. They coaxed Harold to come and meet me. And when he came his face was as red as mine felt. As Harold approached the bench his opening remarks were "We may as well sit together, and make all of these people happy and in so doing, we might find that we are making ourselves happy too."

Harold said he heard that I have a stamp collection and that he also collects stamps. It was obvious that he had been given some information about me. Conversation came easily and we talked incessantly. It was as though we had known each other all of our lives. We sat together until it was time for us to return individually to our quarters. A Wonderful, Wonderful Day! Now I wonder when I will see Harold again.[20]

---

20 Not until 1950 and then Harold comes back into my life again.

Monday, October 27, 1947

Connie has been quite ill and gets pains in her stomach so they took her to the Civic Hospital today. I hope that she is going to be alright.

Saturday, November 8th, 1947

I took a weird feeling in my chest last evening and my respiration went up to sixty. A nurse said that some of them thought that I had suffered a mild heart attack but that Dr. Carmichael told them that my heart is alright. Dr. Carmichael told me to walk to the bathroom two or three times daily now, but to walk very slowly, and hopefully my breathing will improve with increased activity. Since having the surgery in the spring I have been allowed out of bed only once daily.

Thursday, November 20th, 1947

Connie is still in the Civic Hospital so I sent her a wee parcel with a note inside of it.

Friday, December 5th, 1947

Dr. Carmichael has given me permission to get up to wash and have tub baths with assistance from a nurse. Thus it was that I had my first tub bath in nearly nine months and it felt so good.

Thursday, December 11th, 1947

Father Campeau came to visit and it was a joyous occasion. We had not seen him since June. I think that Father is working too hard.

Connie came back from the Civic Hospital. They decided against surgery and she seems to be getting worse and we are all very concerned over her condition.

Friday, December 19th, 1947

Connie died around six o'clock this evening. The priest anointed her as we stood around her bed and united with the priest in reciting the prayers for the dying as she quietly passed away. Later on when we were back in our room and crying Miss Clement came in. "Stop that crying right now. We all have to die some day. So why get so upset?" Miss Clement was expostulating. Moments later two of us rose from our beds simultaneously and headed for the tub room where tears could, as a rule, be shed in peace. However, someone else had beaten us to the crying room. Much to our surprise, Miss Clement stood there sobbing.

Miss Clement tries to keep a stern front but I've known all along the type of person that she really is. Any nurse who will work overtime without pay to give a feverish patient an extra bath or back rub and do numerous other chores is truly a very dedicated person.

Saturday, December 20th, 1947

The Christmas mail is pouring in and I have received many cards and letters. Today I received a parcel from my cousin Marie Hepp who lives in Alberta. We are close in age and exchange letters. And ever since I have been ill Marie always sends me a Christmas gift.

Saturday, December 27th, 1947

We had four days leave for Christmas and I had a lovely time at home with the family. There was a gentle snow falling and all was very peaceful during our drive back to the Sanatorium this evening with Dick Doherty. Dick sang as we drove along. And while he may seem like a member of our family, he can sing, which is something that none of the Rainas can do! Dick had a great time with the wee pair of underwear that I had knit for him and he carried them around in his pocket for a long time.

Tuesday, December 30th, 1947

St. Bonaventure's Church burned down this morning. We all feel sorry for Father Gratton as he is in charge of this parish. He also does a great deal of work for the patients of the Civic Hospital and for us here at the Sanatorium. Fathers Latendresse and Lacroix came to see me as they were in this area to see Father Gratton and to view the ruins of the church. Dr. Carmichael noticed that I have a cold so I can't go home for New Year's.

Wednesday, December 31st, 1947

Most of the girls are gone home for the holiday and Loretta and I are alone. We are planning to have a 'Midnight Party' with the tree lights on etc. And we will eat some goodies. As we intend to sleep early this evening, Loretta has set her alarm for Midnight.

CHAPTER SIXTEEN

LATE FOR THE PARTY

January 1, 1948 – November 11, 1949
Twenty-One Years, Two Months – Twenty-Three Years, One Month

Thursday, January 1ˢᵗ, 1948

Loretta's alarm failed to go off and we didn't wake up until 2:00 a.m. However, we still had our party even though it was a couple of hours late. Imagine a New Year's Party at two o'clock in the morning, in a hospital room with no drinks served, and only two people in attendance! Well, our imaginations made up for everything else that was lacking, so I guess it could be said that the party was a success. We are able to chuckle just by thinking how ridiculous the whole thing was.

Father Bilodeau came and he stayed for a long and enjoyable visit. Dr. Carmichael popped in to wish us a Happy New Year.

Friday, January 16ᵗʰ, 1948

When Dr. Carmichael made rounds he noticed that I was wearing a new pair of pyjamas. Then he went on to give us a blow to blow account of a shopping trip that he had made to buy some nightgowns for his wife. He had to go to several stores before finding exactly what he wanted and the details were quite amusing. Dr. Carmichael always notices the clothes that a person is wearing. And I think that he is the most observant person whom I have ever known. He remarks when we change our hair style and even comments when we change the colour of our lipstick.

Tuesday, January 20th, 1948

Mary came this evening and she brought us a whole barbecued chicken and Mrs. Powers heated some spinach for us. My roommates and I all love chicken and, strange as it may seem, we all like spinach so we had a real feast.

Thursday, February 5th, 1948

Another evening for feasting. Mother came today and she brought a whole roasted chicken.

Wednesday, February 11th, 1948

This is Ash Wednesday and I am going to read the Mass and say the Stations of the Cross every day during Lent.

Tuesday, March 9th, 1948

Father Campeau dropped in and I was delighted to see him. Before Father left I gave him a copy of the Miraculous Medal Magazine with my picture in it that was taken at the Marian Congress last June.

Wednesday, March 24th, 1948

Dr. Carmichael gave me permission to go downstairs to the dining room for my supper every second evening. With the permission went strict orders that I must count to ten on every step when ascending and descending the stairs. The patients are usually allowed up every day when they start going to the dining room. Nevertheless, I am very happy. I might find that every second day is quite enough for me.

Thursday, March 25th, 1948

I had a sputum test this morning and Dr. Carmichael came over this afternoon to tell me that the results are positive G-Seven. This is the highest positive test that I have ever had and I am very disappointed. Dr. Carmichael appeared to be shocked with the results, so that makes the two of us.

Yesterday I was so happy. Why does good news have to be followed with bad news so much of the time?

Sunday, March 28th, 1948

I wasn't allowed to go home and this is Easter Sunday. But I was given permission to attend Mass here and that was a comfort as I had not been to Mass for over a year. Dick Doherty came this afternoon and brought me a box of chocolates. He is a kind and generous person.

Friday, April 2nd, 1948

I walked over to the Whitney Building for a dental checkup and there were at least twelve cavities wanting attention. When is another matter, as dental care is not very speedy around here.

Tuesday, April 6th, 1948

Mary phoned Dr. Carmichael to ask him if he thought that Streptomycin would be beneficial to me and, if so, that she would pay for it. Streptomycin is the new drug being used on a few selected cases of tuberculosis and the patients receiving it must pay for their injections. Dr. Carmichael did not recommend it for me at this time.

Thursday, April 8th, 1948

During the afternoon I was struck with very sharp pains in my stomach and right side. Then I began to vomit. Dr.

Carmichael examined me and before leaving he instructed the nurses to call him if my condition worsened even though he will not be the doctor on call tonight. Mrs. Bryce sent for Dr. Carmichael again at ten o'clock p.m. Upon his arrival he took blood tests and an ice pack was applied to the painful area. Then I was given a hypo for the pain.

Friday, April 9th, 1948

I couldn't sleep last night even though I was given a second hypo. My stomach is still upset and I am only getting boiled water to drink. Dr. Carmichael took more blood tests and he may bring in a surgeon for consultation. However, they don't want to operate unless it becomes absolutely necessary as they do not consider me a good surgical risk. Dr. Carmichael said that I always need longer than the normal time to recover from surgery for illness.

I have suffered from pains in the right side of my stomach at various times since 1942 but have only casually mentioned them to the doctor on one or two occasions before this episode. When I was on exercise in 1942 the pains would become quite severe at times when I was out walking. I mentioned the pains to the doctor at that time and he said there might be some trouble elsewhere in my body besides my chest and that could be why my lung was not progressing satisfactorily in spite of the fact that I was cooperating and obeying all of the rules. At that time the doctor also said that they would check me over from head to toe in an attempt to locate any hidden trouble but first I would have blood tests.

As usually was the case, my sedimentation was very low. Thus no further tests were done. Sometimes I can't help but think that sedimentation rating is one of my worst enemies. I seem to be able to have a lot of medical problems and still come up with a very low sedimentation rate.

Sunday, April 11th, 1948

I am feeling much better and was able to eat soup and ice cream for dinner. However, Dr. Carmichael feels that I might have more of these spells in the future. Personally, I am convinced that there is something quite seriously wrong with my side and has been for several years.

Monday, May 10th, 1948

I had blood tests and my sedimentation is SEVEN. See what I mean about a low sed rate? My last sputum test was 'positive G-Seven' which is extremely bad. Then all those stomach and side pains. Now, this low sedimentation rate. I think that the best part of me is my sedimentation rate. It doesn't make sense and I am baffled.

Thursday, May 20th, 1948

A day to reminisce again. My last day in school was seven years ago today. And the state of my health is much worse now that it was at that time. What a blessing that we cannot see into the future.

Saturday, May 29th, 1948

Mary Brennan is with the Legion of Mary and comes to visit us most Saturday afternoons. These visits have been going on for many years and we like Miss Brennan and look forward to chatting with her. Miss Brennan told us today that she will be going to Ireland for two months and will tell us all about her trip when she returns. I am sure that we will almost feel as though we took this trip with her as she can relate her stories so well. Even though we cannot go on trips, I do love to hear all about the holidays that other people take.

Monday, May 31st, 1948

Dr. Carmichael remarked about the weight that I have lost and that he intends to send me home for a while and let Mother feed me and put some weight on my long skinny neck. The results of having ribs removed from both sides is supposed to be a long skinny neck and the doctors often tease me about that part of my anatomy.

Monday, June 14th, 1948

Clergy day again! We were delighted with a visit from Father Campeau. Then Father Gratton brought his new assistant to meet us. His name is Father Sabourin.

Thursday, July 8th, 1948

The Air Force Band came and played their music on the lawn and this was the first time that I was allowed to attend one of these performances. Thus it was an exciting day for me. Various bands occasionally come to perform for the patients and they enjoy the music.

Wednesday, July 14th, 1948

Once again Dr. Carmichael showed my back to a visiting doctor and explained my thoracoplasty surgery to him.

Saturday, July 31st, 1948

The girls made a farewell party for me as I will be going home tomorrow. Dr. Carmichael was in to say goodbye. And many of the nurses came in to extend their best wishes for a happy holiday at home.

Sunday, August 1st, 1948

Dick Doherty and Earl drove Ralph and me home to Kemptville. Mother was all prepared to receive us and I am happy to be at home. But deep down inside I am sad, as it is the same old story. I am only home for a change in atmosphere but not because I am better. And there are times that I can't help but wish that I could be part of the normal world around me instead of remaining in this cocoon day after day. However, I do try to accept my life as God's will and believe that there must be a reason for all of this. Dear Mother really has the worst deal of all of us, but she is ever loving, patient and kind.

Tuesday, August 10th, 1948

I went to the dentist in Kemptville and had one tooth filled. There are about twelve more cavities so will have several more trips to Dr. Pratt before I am through.

I am enjoying the home cooked meals and feel that I have already gained weight since coming home.

I have gone outside a few times to watch Nick and Jim feeding the calves and milking the cows and have learned to keep my distance. Anne has been the victim of their milk squirting sessions on numerous occasions and it makes such a sticky mess in her hair. The older ones all enjoy Anne and perhaps they do spoil her a wee bit, but she also has to take a lot of teasing. Lou brought a kitten home for Anne and she calls it Oxter. The name is really Oscar but Anne can't pronounce it so everyone is constantly asking about the kitten just to hear the comical way that she says its name.

Friday, August 27th, 1948

Received the first monthly cheque of what is referred to as 'After San Care' and it is for twenty-five dollars. The health nurse came here yesterday for the third time since we came home from the Sanatorium on August 1st.

Saturday, September 4th, 1948

I received an eight page letter from Miss Clement and was so pleased to hear all about what is going on back at the Sanatorium.

Tuesday, September 7th, 1948

Ralph drove me in to Kemptville to visit Noni and we spoke about old times while in the San together. Noni is the girl who made Winganonimous, the praying bear, while we were roommates in the Preventorium.

Monday, September 20th, 1948

I received a letter from Father Campeau and was so happy. His letters give me a great deal of courage that is badly needed to accept this illness more cheerfully.

Saturday, September 25th, 1948

Ralph and Mother took me to church this morning and I went to Confession before Mass. This was the first time that I have received Communion inside a church since that fateful day of May 20th, 1941 and it was a feeling of elation. I prayed for my family and friends but the special intentions of Mass and Communion were offered for my special priest, Father Campeau.

Mary is home for the weekend and she made me a lovely plaid skirt. And the rest of the family bought me a white blouse to go with it.

Monday, October 4th, 1948

Ralph and I were in Ottawa for a checkup and then we went with George to a movie and we had a nice time. After that I had supper with Mary at the Laurentian Terrace where she is staying.

I gained nearly nine pounds since coming home.

Thursday, October 21st, 1948

The family took me to the turkey supper in the Oddfellows Hall that is sponsored annually by Holy Cross Parish. I enjoyed the outing as this gave me an opportunity to meet a number of wonderful people from Kemptville.

Thursday, December 16th, 1948

Most of the family had bad colds with a high fever and I had it too. Now I can't laugh without wheezing. I received a letter from Dr. Carmichael and they may leave me at home for a while longer.

Thursday, December 23rd, 1948

The Christmas mail is coming in and I received a letter from Father Campeau today. He is going to say a Mass for me at Christmas and I think that is one of the nicest gifts that a person can receive.

Wednesday, January 5th, 1949

I sent a get well card to Dr. Carmichael as he has once again undergone surgery and is a patient in the Civic Hospital.

Month of February, 1949

I've had a bad cold for several weeks and I do a lot of wheezing. Also have a sore throat and a large swollen gland on the left side of my neck and am running a fever. The sore neck prevents me from sleeping well at night.

Monday, February 28th, 1949

I had to go to Ottawa today to keep an eye appointment with Dr. Patterson. I was feeling very punk so Dr. Patterson and his nurse had me lie down. They were very kind. This was my first eye examination ever and I will now have to wear glasses for reading.

I also had a checkup at the San today and was looked after by Dr. Jeffrey as Dr. Carmichael is still away on sick leave. Dr. Jeffrey was very concerned over my swollen glands and seems to think that they might be tubercular and warned me not to rub my neck under any circumstances. My temperature was over 102 when I arrived home and I feel very sick.

Easter Sunday, April 17th, 1949

We listened to Father Patrick Peyton's 'Triumphant Hour' on the radio and it was beautiful. Father Peyton has a great love for the Blessed Virgin Mary and I am greatly impressed with the work that he is doing to promote a greater devotion to the Rosary.

Saturday, April 30th, 1949

I received a letter from Dr. Carmichael and after discussing the checkup that I had from Dr. Lloyd two weeks ago, they have decided to allow me to remain at home for the summer. Dr. Carmichael thanked me for the card that I sent him when he was ill.

My neck is better and the swollen glands were not TB after all.

Thursday, June 23rd, 1949

I had worn my hair in braids for years so decided to go to Adele's today and get a permanent for five dollars. This was my first permanent ever and it will take a while getting used to it.

Lou took me to see *The Best Years of Our Lives* in the Kemptville Theatre this evening and it was an excellent movie. The show was about three men returning from the war and the adjustments they had to make after they arrived home. In a way, the movie reminded me of us TB patients because we feel like fish out of water when we are discharged from the Sanatorium and our adjustments are also very difficult to make.

Friday, July 1st, 1949

Mary is home on holidays and working like a beaver to surprise Mother when she comes home from the hospital. Mary papered and painted the parlour and it looks so nice. Then Lou and Mary bought linoleum for the dining room and it looks great.

Friday, July 8th, 1949

Mother came home after spending five weeks in the hospital for surgery. We are all very excited but I think that Dad is the happiest one of all as he really missed Mother.

Mom was very surprised when she saw the new linoleum and all the other things that the family had done while she was away.

Tuesday, September 6th, 1949

Anne, the youngest member of our large family, started to school today and she likes it. We are all interested in hearing about Anne's experiences in school and on the bus.

Tuesday, September 13th, 1949

When Jimmy came home from school today he was greeted by three chattering squirrels scurrying around on top of the kitchen roof and the sight of them way up there was very upsetting to our youngest brother. Jimmy had cared for these squirrels since their infancy. He had fed them warm milk out of Anne's wee doll bottle and watched over them like a mother hen. Then we all grieved for Jimmy when two squirrels died and rejoiced with him as the other three progressed into healthy pets. When they became more active Jimmy built a large wooden cage for them outside. We enjoyed their antics and no one gave much thought about their future and what their teeth would be able to do. Well today was their day of reckoning. They chewed their way to freedom and were enjoying it immensely. But Jimmy was distraught so Louis tried to recapture the pets for him and received a nasty bite on his finger. The squirrels let it be known that they were not about to be recaptured. After watching the squirrels fighting for their freedom, Jimmy realized that his pets could no longer be kept captive and he was able to accept and to understand that this is the way it should be.[21]

More September news, 1949

The Waterworks were turned on in the Town of Kemptville. This was a big event.

And Dick Doherty entered the Seminary to become a priest. I hope that he will be very happy. He is a generous person and has been very kind to our family.

Saturday, September 24th, 1949

Mother and Mary combined together and purchased a lovely new green coat for me at a cost of $39.50. This is the first coat ever that was bought for me so needless to say I am very excited. However, I did get one other new coat before now. Mother made me a little blue coat when I was about four years old and I can still remember the buttons that were on it. I can also remember the first time that I wore that coat. Mother had

---

21 These three squirrels remained close to home for many weeks but no one was ever able to capture them again.

baked meringues for us children to eat while travelling in the back of the wagon and I was very cautious so as not to soil my pretty new coat. Mother says that my eyes and the coat were exactly the same shade of blue.

Thursday, October 6th, 1949

About three weeks ago Lou bought a 1930 Chevrolet car and he paid $250.00 cash for it. Since Louis has a car, Mary and Lou decided that they would take me to Montreal for my birthday. We left early this morning and enjoyed the trip while driving along the St. Lawrence River. We went to a movie this evening and then we settled down for the night.

Friday, October 7th, 1949

This morning we took a Scenic Bus Tour of Montreal which included several interesting stops. We visited the church of Notre Dame, the Wax Works, St. Joseph's Oratory and Brother André's room.

Saturday, October 8th, 1949

We left Montreal early this morning and came back through Alexandria so we could visit Sister St. Mildred in the convent there. Sister had taught both Lou and me at Billings Bridge and she was pleased to see us.

I was tired by the time we arrived home but it was a wonderful birthday present and I am happy.

Sunday, October 16th, 1949

I went to Confession, received Holy Communion and attended Mass this morning and once again had a feeling of elation after being in church.

Wednesday, October 19th, 1949

I am very tired. I've just had nearly three days of pain in the right side of my stomach again. Dr. Beamish came a few times to give me hypos and pills. He was very tempted to send me to the Civic Hospital for surgery. I've awakened with pain at least once every night for the past several months and I have lost quite a bit of weight.

Thursday, November 10th, 1949

I am trying to put my room and all of my belongings in order as I do not feel well. I am suffering so much with the pains in my side and feel certain that I cannot go on much longer this way and will end up dying unless they operate on me.

Friday, November 11th, 1949

We went to see *Bambi* at the theatre and we even managed to get Dad to come with us to celebrate his birthday.

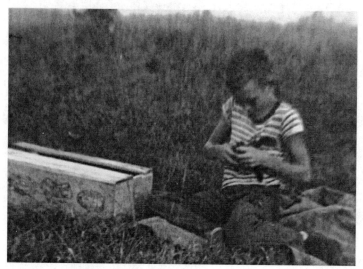

Summer 1949, Kemptville, Ontario.
Jimmy with his squirrels.

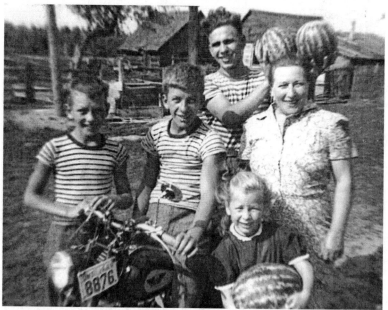

On our farm at Kemptville, Ontario.
L to R: Jimmy, Nicky, Mother (Elizabeth Raina)
Back: Louis   *Front:* Anne

CHAPTER SEVENTEEN

MORE SURGERY

November 14, 1949 – March 7, 1950
Twenty-Three Years, One Month – Twenty-Three Years, Five Months

Monday, November 14th, 1949

I was very sick all night and never knew until now that it was possible to suffer so much pain. However, I never told anyone that I was ill until this morning. Then Mother phoned Dr. Beamish and he came to see me and was very kind. This time he made immediate arrangements for me to enter the Civic Hospital.

John O'Neill very kindly drove Mother and me to Ottawa and I was relieved when I was settled in bed again. I was lying down on the back seat of the car on the way in and all the while eagerly waiting to see a doctor and be in a hospital bed.

Doctor Max Vechter is looking after me and he made arrangements for me to be operated on at eight o'clock this evening. Father Campeau came to see me and to hear my Confession and now I feel quite calm and am not too worried about what lies ahead. In fact, I think there is a tremendous feeling of relief just knowing that now the cause of all these pains might be discovered.

Tuesday, November 15th, 1949

Father Campeau waited on the bench with Mother and Mary during the entire operation and when I awoke the three of them were at my bedside. Father Campeau returned again early this morning and gave me Holy Communion.

Shortly after I was wheeled in for surgery Dr. Hermann recognized Mother as he was passing by so he went into the operating room and watched most of the operation.

Dr. Carmichael dropped in to see me this morning and he asked me if they had run off with my appendix and I automatically answered "Yes." After Dr. Carmichael was gone I suddenly realized that I haven't a clue yet as to what the operation was about.

Thursday, November 17th, 1949

My stomach is still upset and I am very weak. Dr. Vechter sent the dietician in to see me and I was told to ask for whatever I feel like eating. I am getting Vitamin B injections and hope that they will help me.

Dr. Vechter is taking excellent care of me and promised that he will explain the nature of my operation when I am stronger. I suspect that I either had TB or cancer but most likely TB.

A patient from one of the other rooms came in and started asking questions. When I wasn't able to tell her what type of surgery I had she came to her own conclusions. She said that when the doctor withholds information it usually means cancer.

Yesterday Dr. Hermann stopped in for a wee chat and I was so pleased to see him. He said that my right fallopian tube was very bad and that I must have suffered a great deal. Maybe they had to remove the tube. I don't know.

Dr. Carmichael dropped in again this morning while on his way to work. He said that he will be back again. I have a feeling that he wants to tell me that I will be returning to the Sanatorium when I leave the Civic Hospital.

Monday, November 21st, 1949

Doctor Dave Roger dropped in to see me and this pleased me very much. And the nurses from the Sanatorium have not forgotten me. Miss Clement, Mrs. Powers and little Miss Walker have all been here to see me.

Father Campeau comes often and the patients think so highly of him. He is so understanding of the needs of the sick.

Dr. Vechter comes to see me every day and gives the very best of care. He is an excellent doctor. At least I know that is what I think of him.

Tuesday, November 22nd, 1949

Dr. Dave Roger's wife and his mother came to visit and they brought me a lovely bouquet of flowers. This was the first time that I met Dr. Roger's wife and she is a very charming lady. I was so pleased with the visit from these two lovely ladies.

Rita O'Neill came last evening and her mother was here today. Rita is John O'Neill's sister and the O'Neill family are very good neighbours of ours at Kemptville. Barbara Lecuyer has also been here to see me and she is always so pleasant.

Thursday, November 24th, 1949

Dr. Carmichael came to see me and just as I suspected, he wants me to go back into the Sanatorium. Actually, I am relieved, though sad, as I really do feel much too sick and weak to be going home.

Friday, November 25th, 1949

Dr. Vechter came this afternoon and just as promised, he explained the nature of my surgery to me. The appendix and both fallopian tubes were removed. The right tube was greatly enlarged and indicated ample reason for causing severe pains. The left tube was also affected and had to be removed. Tuberculosis was involved and it was also removed. The operation was absolutely necessary but as the result of it, I never will be able to have any children.

I know this would have come as a great blow except that when I had thoracoplasty surgery on my second side I was given stiff warnings never to become pregnant. I was cautioned that with both lungs collapsed at the top, my breathing is mostly done with the movement of my stomach muscles, thus making it impossible to carry a child full term so I never could give birth to a living child.

Being Roman Catholic, and not wanting to break the rules of my Religion, I have always just taken it more or less for granted that I never would be able to get married.

Saturday, November 26th, 1949

I was supposed to be transferred to the Sanatorium today but I had a serious relapse. My stomach was very upset, my pulse was weak and irregular and I had pains in my left side. Dr. Vechter was in several times alone and with another doctor. Dr. Vechter phoned Dr. Carmichael to tell him that my transfer will be delayed. Fathers Campeau and Gratton were here today.

Monday, November 28th, 1949

Dr. Carmichael came to tell me that I will be transferred by ambulance to the Sanatorium tomorrow and I will be put into the Whitney Building. They want to have me close to the doctors so they can keep a watchful eye on me in case I have another relapse like the one I had on Saturday.

I am very disappointed. I wanted to be in the Preventorium Building with Miss Clement and all of my other friends. I will try to accept this as God's will but it will be very, very difficult.

Father Gratton brought us Communion again this morning and I get a great comfort from my religion. I am always so pleased when the priests bring us Holy Communion.

Tuesday, November 29th, 1949

Father Campeau came this afternoon just before I was transferred to the Sanatorium by Veitch Ambulance. It was a great comfort so see Father as I was extremely blue.

Now I am with two other women, in Room 10B, Second Floor, Whitney Building. I have seldom felt this blue before. I wanted to be in the Preventorium. And I miss home! Anne is a delightful and interesting little sister. She used to come in early every morning and close my window so the room would be warm when I got out of bed. Jimmy is such a lovable tease with a great sense of humour. Mother is one of the best parents in the whole world. Every member of the family has his or her own wonderful traits and how I miss each and every one of them.

And how I miss home! I sure need God's help now.

Monday, December 12th, 1949

Dr. Lloyd examined me and he can hear râles on both sides of my chest so he doesn't know where the positive sputum is coming from. My weight is down to 105 pounds and my Vital Capacity is 36%. They will discuss giving me Streptomycin.

Wednesday, December 14th, 1949

Dr. Lloyd ordered Streptomycin and PAS for a period of sixty days. I will get two Streptomycin injections daily as well as four PAS pills. I sure hope that these drugs will help me.

Sunday, December 18th, 1949

My sister Mary and Dick Doherty were in to see me. Dick is on three weeks leave from the Seminary. He joked about me going to Confession but I can't imagine ever confessing to him. However, I do think that he will be a very good priest. It's just because we grew up together that I feel this way about going to Confession to him.

Wednesday, December 28th, 1949

Dr. Carmichael is very ill and was taken to Montreal for surgery. We were told that Dr. Wilder Penfield operated to remove a blood clot from Dr. Carmichael's brain. I am very worried so am praying hard for Dr. Carmichael's recovery.

Thursday, December 29th, 1949

Miss Pearl Walker made rounds this morning and said that Dr. Carmichael had phoned to say that he is fine and sends his love to everyone. That is wonderful news.

Saturday, December 31st, 1949

Father Bilodeau came to visit and gave us his blessing for the New Year.

Sunday, January 1st, 1950

Father Campeau brought us Communion. I really don't know what I would do without Father to keep my spirits up as I find the Whitney Building is so depressing and I am constantly wishing that I was in the Preventorium again.

Wednesday, January 25th, 1950

I came back to the Preventorium today and I am elated. I am in Room Eight with three girls whom I have known for a long time; Denise, Maureen and Doris.

Monday, February 13th, 1950

Dr. Carmichael is back working part time and I saw him today when I was over at the Whitney for x-rays. He was in a good mood and we had a nice chat.

In some ways I suppose I am very lucky. I have good parents and a good family at home. Here at the Sanatorium there is Dr. Carmichael, Miss Clement and Father Campeau. They are very good to me and I think of them as 'The Three Great Cs'.

Wednesday, March 1st, 1950

The nurses will occasionally ask me to do some little job for them. And today they brought in a pillow slip full of stockings to sort and darn for the younger children. There is enough work here to keep me out of mischief for a while.

Tuesday, March 7th, 1950

Mary Brennan brought me a bag full of stamps for my stamp collection and I am delighted with them. Now I have something else to keep me busy for a few more days.

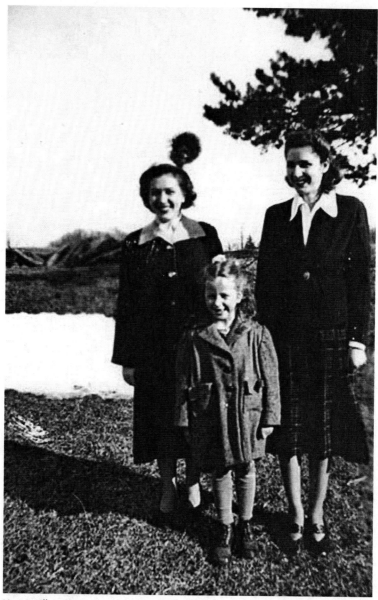

Kemptville, Ontario. The Three Raina Sisters
Left to Right: Mary, Anne, Clara

CHAPTER EIGHTEEN

HAROLD COMES BACK INTO MY LIFE AGAIN

March 10, 1950 – March 28, 1950
Twenty-Three Years, Five Months

Friday, March 10th, 1950

Happy, Happy Day! I should be writing this in coloured ink so it would stand out.

Remember Harold? He is the gentleman who I used to watch from my window in 1947. We have not seen each other since that day when we sat together on the lawn bench in October of 1947. I have thought about Harold at various times but tried to wipe the memories from my mind as I never expected to see him again and assumed that he had forgotten all about me.

Today Harold sent me some candy and nuts with another patient who came to visit at the Preventorium. Harold is waiting to have a thoracoplasty operation and is supposed to cut down on goodies until after the surgery. I conveyed my thanks through this other patient but would like to write and thank Harold personally only I do not want it to look as though I am chasing after him. This has been a wonderful day!

Tuesday, March 28th, 1950

Dr. Lloyd examined me and he couldn't hear nearly as many râles on my chest so he was very pleased. And my stomach lavage and sputum tests are all negative now. However, Dr. Lloyd cautioned "Don't get too excited as we don't know how long these good things will last."

CHAPTER NINETEEN

A VISIT FROM THE GRAND JURY

April 5, 1950 – December 31, 1950
Twenty-Three Years, Six Months – Twenty-Four Years, Two Months

Wednesday, April 5th, 1950

It is customary for the Grand Jury to make a periodic inspection of the institutions in the Ottawa area and then a report of their findings will appear in an Ottawa paper on the following day. No one ever knows the day or the time when these men will put in their appearance. And this year they seem to be more critical than usual and have had some unfavourable remarks published about certain institutions. We all know that Dr. Carmichael is doing a tremendous job of running the Sanatorium and we also know that he would be deeply hurt if there were any unfavourable remarks published about our hospital. Thus we waited in nervous anticipation for our turn to come.

And then today was our day of reckoning. Dr. Carmichael led these men (twelve I think) into our room and his opening remarks were "Clara, I was telling these men about all the ribs that you have out of both sides and they can't understand what is holding you together. So will you please sit up and let me show them your back?" As I bared my back to these men I was very thankful that they were all strangers and not our next door neighbours. After looking at my back, these men began to ask questions. "What type of work will she be able to do when she is discharged from the Sanatorium?" "Clara is just waiting to go home and help out on the farm" responded Dr. Carmichael.

Then Dr. Carmichael hastily left the room and moved on to the next selected case. However, two of these men did not follow the doctor out but remained to ask more questions. "What type of farm work could I do? Did I drive a tractor?"

As they put words into my mouth I would answer, "Yes, I drove the tractor" and so on. The truth is that I cannot drive a tractor nor a car and can barely tell the front end of a vehicle from its rear end. Those were tense moments and my roommates signalled with crossed fingers from their beds that were situated behind the backs of these two men. The nurses and patients all chuckled a little after Dr. Carmichael and his entourage had left the Preventorium in spite of our concern for tomorrow's paper.

Thursday, April 6th, 1950

We eagerly awaited the arrival of the newspaper today so we could read what the Grand Jury had to say about the Sanatorium. And what a relief! It is a glowing report and everyone is extremely happy.

Thursday, April 13th, 1950

Harold had his first stage of thoracoplasty surgery today and I am praying that he will be all right. I sent him a get well card and thanked him for the goodies that he gave me a while ago.

Sunday, April 16th, 1950

I heard that Harold's father died yesterday and hope this won't cause a set back in his recovery. I am praying for the repose of Mr. Mouré's soul and for Harold.

Friday, April 22nd, 1950

I had a very pleasant surprise. I received my first letter from Harold and I am so happy.

Friday, May 5th, 1950

I received another letter from Harold. He wrote it yesterday before he went down for his second stage surgery. I am praying very hard so that he will be all right.

Wednesday, May 24th, 1950

I wasn't allowed to attend the movie shown at the Whitney Building this evening and I am very disappointed as the other patients had it all arranged that Harold and I would sit together.

Tuesday, May 30th, 1950

Simone and I have said our beads together every day during the month of May. Dick Doherty is home on holidays from the Seminary and it is so nice to visit with him again.

Wednesday, June 21st, 1950

Dr. Carmichael has given me permission to go to the dining room for supper. And as the rule now stands, patients with dining room privileges also have lawn privileges so I am looking forward to a very exciting summer.

Monday, June 26th, 1950

My sputum tests are all negative. My sedimentation is four and my haemoglobin is 89%. Dr. Carmichael said I might be able to go home in August.

Sunday, July 16th, 1950

Dr. Lloyd has given me permission to visit my brothers Ralph and George at the Perley on Sunday afternoons and while I was there today I saw Harold. He is so wonderful!

Tuesday, July 18th, 1950

I received a letter from Mother and she told me that Dad has tuberculosis and will have to enter the Sanatorium. Poor Dad and poor Mother too. I feel so sorry for both of them.

Father Campeau was here and he is going to pray for Dad.

Saturday, July 22nd, 1950

Mackenzie King died.

Saturday, July 29th, 1950

Dr. Carmichael told me that I won't be able to go home next month as planned since Dad is sick and will have to enter the Sanatorium. I was tempted to tell Dr. Carmichael that I am needed to help out on the farm and to drive the tractor.

Father Campeau took several of us for a drive to Quenel's Bowling Alley and while we were there he bought us all ice cream cones.

Sunday, July 30th, 1950

Father Campeau said Mass here this morning.

I had a pleasant chat with Harold when I was visiting Ralph at the Perley this afternoon. Dick Doherty was also here visiting and when visiting hour was over he accompanied me back to the Preventorium. Dick had seen me speaking with Harold and I don't think that he approves of our friendship. Not that he has anything against Harold but because a romance could interfere with the relationship that exists between God and me.

Friday, August 18th, 1950

I saw Harold dressed in street clothes for the first time and he looked so distinguished as he stood there by the gate. Previously he was always attired in his dressing gown. Harold was put up for one meal a week ago and I am very happy for him. I wish that we were in the same building so we could see each other more often.

Thursday, August 24th, 1950

Louis brought us some corn on the cob and it was still deliciously warm after coming all the way in from Kemptville. Once again Mother had wrapped it in several layers of newspaper over waxed paper which seems to be the best way of keeping food warm for a long period of time.

Friday, August 25th, 1950

This was the day for the yearly Ottawa Exhibition special Grandstand Performance at Lansdowne Park that is put on for the elderly, the orphans and the shut-ins. The performers do their acts free of charge. And the drivers who take us to and from Lansdowne Park donate their time as well as the use of their cars. There were about a hundred and twenty patients from the Sanatorium alone to transport both ways and there were many other institutions to look after as well. Thus we can just surmise that this very successful event was the result of many hard working and generous individuals. We appreciate their generosity and I will always remember today.

Generally the patients who go together sit together at the Grandstand Performance so when Harold came over to speak with me through the window last evening, I got all excited as

I thought sure that he came to ask me to sit with him. But no such luck! He wanted to tell me that he had promised to look after an elderly gentleman. He would sit with him in the front row and give him his undivided attention. This gent had been through a rough time and Harold felt that the outing would do him the world of good. My first reaction was a feeling of great disappointment and even anger but I refrained from verbally expressing my emotions. However, Harold's offer to look after the elderly gent fits right in with all that I have heard about him, ever thoughtful and kind.

After the performance today I had the opportunity to speak briefly with Harold and his elderly charge. This old gent was glowing as he spoke of Harold's kindness for looking after him. Seeing the happiness that this gentleman was experiencing made me realize, more than ever, just how wonderful Harold is. And it was as though Harold's eyes were asking me to understand why he had volunteered to look after this man and to share in the satisfaction that resulted from this deed.

Now I do realize more than ever just how wonderful Harold really is and my interest in him continues to grow.

Monday, August 28th, 1950

My sister Mary and Dick were here this evening and I was lonesome after they left. Dick's holidays are over and he will be leaving for the Seminary in the States and it will probably be a year until we see him again.

Saturday, September 2nd, 1950

When Dr. Carmichael made rounds he sat on my bed and showed me some pictures that were taken at our picnic of 1943. We did a good job of remembering the names of the people in his photos.

Tuesday, September 12th, 1950

Yesterday I wrote a letter to Father Patrick Peyton and invited him to visit us while he is in Ottawa next week.[22] After the letter was mailed some of the patients said that I should have obtained Dr. Carmichael's permission before extending the invitation to Father Peyton. Then an incident from the past flashed through my mind and that sure didn't help matters.

A roommate of mine had once written to Barbara Ann Scott, the skater, and invited her to come and visit us girls in the Preventorium. The next thing we knew, Dr. Carmichael came into our room and he was not in his usual jovial mood. He had just received a phone call from Prime Minister Mackenzie King who was speaking on behalf of Barbara Ann Scott. Mackenzie King did not appreciate the invitation. He said that Barbara Ann was still a young girl and was in need of plenty of rest and could not be going around to visit patients inside hospitals etc. We never could figure out why Prime Minister Mackenzie King was responding to a letter that had been written to the skater herself!

Thus the more I thought about the letter written to Father Peyton the more worried I became. Suddenly I decided that I would speak to Harold about my problems. He had come to the

---

22 "During Father Peyton's final year in the seminary he was diagnosed with tuberculosis, considered incurable at that time. He was given little hope by the medical team of recovering to full health. Fr Patrick had great faith and prayed to the Blessed Virgin Mary for a recovery to health. His prayers were answered and his health began to improve to the amazement of the medical profession. He was ordained to the priesthood on June 15, 1941. "Father Patrick Peyton – The Rosary Priest – Peyton Memorial Centre, http://www.museumsofmayo.com/peyton1.htm, 23/08/2010. " The formal declaration of the opening of the diocesan phase of the canonization process for Father Patrick Peyton was announced on June 1, 2001 in Fall River, Mass, a few days after receiving approval from the Vatican's Congregation for the Causes of the Saints." HCFM: Sainthood: Current Status, http://www.hcfm.org/main/cause.php, 23/08/2010. (Clara would have been so happy to hear of the canonization process for Father Peyton).

window with Ralph this morning and said that he would return to visit me when I was out on the lawn this afternoon.

When I told Harold about my predicament he made it all sound so simple and immediately put my mind at rest. He suggested that I get a letter right off in the mail to Father Campeau explaining what I had done. Father Campeau is our Chaplain and Harold said that he will know what to do.

Well I did exactly as Harold had suggested and mailed a letter to Father Campeau. Now I am breathing much easier again.

Tuesday, September 19th, 1950

Father Campeau came this morning to pass the word around that Father Patrick Peyton will be speaking to the patients this afternoon in the waiting room at the Whitney Building.

We had just assembled at the waiting room when Father Campeau motioned for me to come out into the hall. Father Peyton was there and he said that he wanted to meet me so he could personally thank me for the lovely letter that I had written to him. This was an emotional experience as I felt that I was shaking hands with a future Saint.

Father Peyton was so humble and sincere as he spoke to us that I felt he surely must be one of the Blessed Virgin Mary's favourite persons. Then as he told of his miraculous cure from tuberculosis the sincerity of his words seemed to ooze out of every pore of his body and it was a very memorable and moving experience for me.

After Father Peyton's departure Harold walked back to the Pre with me and we sat on the bench and talked until it was time for each of us to return to our respective buildings.

Later this evening I kept thinking about Father Peyton and the impression that he made on me. Until now I have always enjoyed reading about the lives of the Saints as I was forever searching for clues to find out if other people knew it when they were living in the presence of a real Saint and how it would feel to meet this living Saint. I suppose that I was always searching for my living Saint and now the hunt is over. I think that Father Peyton is my living Saint and now my great curiosity has been satisfied.

This has been one of the happiest days of my life. Firstly, Father Campeau rescued me from the possibility of a confrontation with Dr. Carmichael. Next there was the meeting with Father Peyton, my living Saint. And then there was the wonderful visit that I had with Harold.

Friday, September 29th, 1950

I was sitting alone on the bench outside and Harold came over and sat with me. I usually see him every day now. Every moment spent with Harold is like a moment in Heaven. I don't think that it would be possible to experience greater happiness than what I feel when I am with Harold. He is so kind and is a perfect gentleman. And he is very religious but has a great sense of humour and is not a bit stuffy. We are never stuck for words and his conversations are always interesting. I think that he is the perfect man, better than my imagination could ever dream up and there is nothing about him that I would want to change.

Sunday, October 1st, 1950

When I was visiting Ralph and Harold at the Perley this afternoon an ex-patient came to visit and she brought me a bouquet of flowers. Harold put the flowers in water to keep them fresh until I returned to the Preventorium and I gave him a carnation from the bouquet to wear in his buttonhole. Just then Jerry, an ex-patient walked into the room and gave Harold quite a teasing about girls and flowers. Jerry has quite a sense of humour and is very generous with his visits to the sick.

Tuesday, October 3rd, 1950

Our lawn privileges have been discontinued but the Perley patients still have theirs so Harold came to the window and I was delighted to see him.

Wednesday, October 4th, 1950

We were given permission to attend the movie at the Whitney this evening and Harold popped over there after the show and told me that their lawn privileges have also been discontinued. Now I don't know when we will be able to see each other again.

Friday, October 13th, 1950

Dad was admitted into the Perley Building today and I hope that he will be able to adjust to life in the Sanatorium.

Thursday, October 26th, 1950

Dr. Carmichael put me up for ten minutes of daily exercise. I haven't been on exercise since 1942 so it certainly will be strange walking down the street again. I am very happy. This has been a great day. My sedimentation rate is three.

Saturday, November 11th, 1950

This is Dad's birthday so the family got together and bought a watch as a gift for him. Now that I am up on exercise I can get over to visit my Father more often. This also gives me the opportunity to visit with Harold in the workshop.

Tuesday, November 21st, 1950

My last sputum tests were positive again after being negative for nine months so Dr. Carmichael put me on another course of Streptomycin and PAS.

Friday, December 1st, 1950

I was on my way to the workshop hoping to see Harold when I heard him calling to me from a window of the Perley Building. He wanted to let me know that he would not be going to the workshop today as he had fainted this morning after having two teeth extracted.

Monday, December 11th, 1950

Dr. Carmichael entered the workshop when Harold and I were speaking to each other and he greeted us in a friendly way without making any snide remarks. They are so quick to say something when a 'San Romance' is suspected as that is a 'no no' around here. The doctors' favourite quote is "Love and TB just don't mix."

Perhaps they just don't suspect that Harold and I care for each other as neither one of us has ever been involved in a San Romance before even though we have both been here for several years. Harold must appeal to everyone as no one seems to worry when they see us together. And there really is no cause for worry as we are not breaking any rules, other than wanting to see each other.

Friday, December 15th, 1950

I am overjoyed! Harold was put up on exercise. And my exercise will increase to fifteen minutes. Now we can take our walks together.

Sunday, December 31st, 1950

I have had a bad cold since coming back from four days at home over the Christmas holidays. Since then I have stayed inside so I will be well enough to go with Harold to my sister Mary's tomorrow. However, I did go over to the Perley today to see Dad and to make the final arrangements with Harold for tomorrow. He will pick me up around two-thirty in the afternoon.

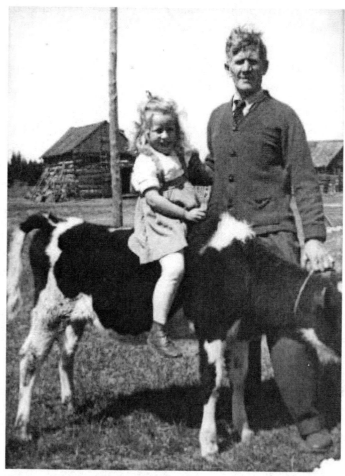

Anne Raina and her father, Dominic Raina, taken at Kemptville, Ontario, summer 1947

CHAPTER TWENTY

HAPPY, HAPPY NEW YEAR

January 1, 1951 – December 31, 1951
Twenty-Four Years, Three Months – Twenty-Five Years,
Two Months

Monday, January 1ˢᵗ, 1951

Harold came for me at two-thirty and we took a taxi to St. Joseph's Church and then we went inside the church to make a visit and to say some prayers. I was so pleased when Harold asked me if I would like to stop off at church as I had been thinking the very same thing but hesitated to ask.

My dream had always been that if ever I met a man that I really cared for that we would make a visit inside a church on our first date. Since this was the first time together away from the Sanatorium I considered this was really our first date or at least our first opportunity to make the all-important church visit of my dream become a reality. I felt that if we remembered God on our first date that God would always remember us. I prayed very fervently and I asked God to always watch over us so we will ever do what is right.

I was filled with wonderful emotions as we left the church and walked the short distance to Mary's apartment on Nelson Street. I knew that I loved God very much and I also felt certain that I loved Harold too.

Mary had prepared a delicious meal and we had a happy time at her place. Then we checked back into the Sanatorium at nine-thirty p.m. and I thanked God for the wonderful day that I had.

Tuesday, January 2nd, 1951

I still have a cold so didn't go out but Harold came to the window to ask how I was.

Saturday, January 6th, 1951

Ralph was put on exercise today so the four of us went for a walk together and we had an hilarious time. The foursome consisted of Ralph, Harold, a friend of mine and me. I see Harold every day unless there is some good reason why we cannot see each other.

Wednesday, January 10th, 1951

Phyllis' mother drove us to see the crib in St. Francis Church and I really appreciated this opportunity as there are many people and things to pray for. However, it meant that I did not get to see Harold today and I missed him. We always enjoy our walks whether it is just the two of us, or four of us, or a whole gang promenading down the street, two by two.

Saturday, January 13th, 1951

There is a new building going up here at the Sanatorium and since all construction ceases on Saturdays, our gang decided to explore the inside of the building this afternoon instead of going on exercise. We tried to guess what each room will be used for when the building is completed. And we even picked out our favourite rooms that we hope to occupy if ever we have to be patients in this building. We had an exciting time as we conquered the numerous obstacles that we encountered on our tour.[23] We took pictures after our tour so today's adventures could long be remembered.

Saturday, January 27th, 1951

When Harold and I were on exercise today I thought our conversation was very interesting as well as being a little bit humorous. Harold told me that he knows people think of him as being old fashioned. He said they probably say "He isn't modernized yet." But that that is the way he is, that he looks before he jumps off the front verandah. Old fashioned or not, I know that I love him just the way that he is and there is not one thing about him that I would want to change. There are times that I try to find something about Harold that is not to my liking as I do not know how I could bear it if we ever broke up. But all I ever end up doing is finding more and more things about him that I do like.

Tuesday, January 30th, 1951

Ralph gave me a lovely black leather purse that he made and I am delighted with it. The patients can buy leather at the workshop and some do quite a bit of leather work and then they sell their finished products. Ralph and George have both occupied quite a bit of their time in this manner.

Wednesday, January 31st, 1951

I went on exercise thinking that I would meet Harold as usual when another chap came along and said that Harold had gone to his uncle's funeral and had asked him to look after me for him. Then this chap delivered many comical messages that supposedly came from Harold but we all knew differently and everyone chuckled at the performance he gave.

---

23 This new building was later christened The Carmichael Building in honour of Dr. Carmichael.

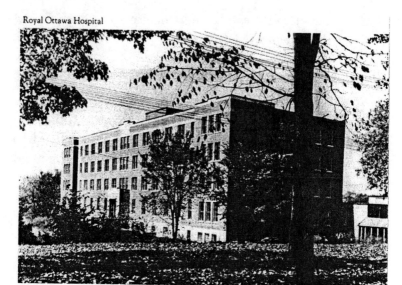

Royal Ottawa Hospital

The Infirmary Building opened in 1953.
The name was later changed to the Carmichael Building.

Friday, February 2nd, 1951

Father Campeau came for Confession and Communion and I was very pleased as I have now completed my 'nine first Fridays.' That means that I have received Communion on the First Friday of nine consecutive months.

Wednesday, February 28th, 1951

Harold and I always wait for each other to take our walks but today Harold just marched on ahead with one of the other chaps. However, when he reached the drug store he stopped and waited for me and we walked back together. Harold said that he was fed up and wasn't fit company for anyone in this frame of mind. He had had a checkup early in February and was told at that time that if all the tests were favourable he would be going home. Now it is weeks later and he is still waiting for the results. This was the first time that I have ever seen Harold angry or heard him complain and I couldn't blame him. I feel sorry for him and I do understand how he feels.

Tuesday, March 13th, 1951

Lou and Nick are joining the Air Force and were in Ottawa today for their medicals.

Ralph went home for good and we are going to miss him on our walks. Harold walked me right back to the Preventorium this afternoon. Maybe he thinks that I am feeling a little lonesome because Ralph went home.

This winter has been the very happiest time in my life. Since I met Harold I have been happier than I ever knew it was possible to be.

Saturday, March 24th, 1951

When Harold and I were out walking this afternoon we met Dr. Carmichael in his car and he just smiled and waved to us. When we first saw his car approaching, we were sure that we would get a disapproving look so that was a relief. We all know how strongly Dr. Carmichael objects to 'San Romances' so perhaps he thinks as some other people do, that Harold and I probably recite our beads while out walking. None of the staff seem to take us seriously except for Miss W., a nurse.

Miss W. had first spotted Harold and me together while looking out of her bedroom window from the nurses' residence. That evening when she came on duty she was bursting with excitement. She said she hoped that I cared for Harold more than just as a casual friend. As Miss W.'s excitement mounted she continued to say that in all the time that she has known Harold and me that she never could imagine Harold with any of the other girls nor me with any of the other men in the Sanatorium. But when she noticed the two of us together she immediately thought of us as the perfect match. She said we were so much alike and she could just vision us being very happy together. Miss W. was so enthused and eager that she even promised that she will give us a nice gift if we get married.

Tuesday, March 27th, 1951

Ralph, Mother, Nick, Jim and Anne came today and it was great seeing so many members of the family. Nick will be leaving this coming Sunday for St. Jean, Quebec, as that is where he will be starting his career in the Air Force.

Tuesday, April 3rd, 1951

Harold took me to the Civic Tea Room for a hot chocolate when we were on our exercise this afternoon. He takes me for a hot chocolate nearly every day. Life is wonderful! Harold had an exam yesterday and if all is well he is supposed to go home in two weeks.

Thursday, April 5th, 1951

Harold and I had another wonderful visit while out on our walk this afternoon. I will miss him so much when he goes home but Dr. Carmichael told me a while back that I will be going home on May 24th if all goes well.

Friday, April 6th, 1951

Father Campeau brought us Communion for the First Friday so the day started out just fine. Then this afternoon I went to the Perley to visit Dad and from there I went on exercise. I met Harold on Carling Avenue and we walked back together. And as we strolled along I became aware of being very short of breath and wondered what was causing this discomfort. Then I decided that we were probably in store for a big change in the weather and that that was my problem.

However, my problem turned out to be much more serious than a weather forecast this time. About two hours after supper I took a coughing spell and haemorrhaged from my left lung. I was given calcium to drink and Dr. Kubilius also injected calcium intravenously into my arm.

Then for the second time in my life I cried in the presence of a doctor. And I do not like crying in front of the doctors and I also know how foolish it is to cry while haemorrhaging from the lungs but I was beyond control of myself today.

Dr. Kubilius was very kind and did his best to comfort me. He said there were many tears shed for me so that I need not cry for myself. All my friends were congregated in a back room and they were crying because I had taken the haemorrhage. I was wondering where my roommates and everyone else had disappeared to.

Every time the tears were about to stop another thought would pop into my mind and then I would start all over again. I thought about Harold. Now I won't be able to see him. What if he gets a new girl friend? What if this and what if that? Questions and more questions? I was given a hypo and Dr. Kubilius did all that he could do for me before leaving. This is such a big cross that God has sent to me!

Saturday, April 7th, 1951

Much of my time last night and today was spent weeping. And I still find it very difficult to accept this latest setback. Every attempt to pray ends in failure as I just cry every time that I try to say "Thy Will Be Done."

The girls said that Harold felt very badly when told that I had haemorrhaged. He came to the window and waved to me even though he knew that I wouldn't be able to speak to him. My heart aches and I sorely missed my walk with Harold today.

Sunday, April 8th, 1951

Another haemorrhage this morning and I feel so weak and sick. Dr. Shemanski came over twice to see me and everyone is so good, especially Miss Clement.

Harold wrote me a lovely letter which helps so much. He is wonderful. God bless him. However, I cry when I see Harold going on exercise because I can't be with him. I am still trying to accept this setback as God's will but find it VERY, VERY difficult.

Wednesday, April 11th, 1951

I am getting my meal trays again but all the food has to be cold before I can eat it. It really feels as though God has forsaken me. And more than anything else I would like to see Father Campeau. I am sure that he could make me see the bright side of life again but I know how busy he is so dare not ask the nurse to send for him. Waiting for Father Campeau's next visit is so hard to bear. This is another golden opportunity to gain merits. If only I could pray? I want to pray but the words won't come – only tears.

Friday, April 13th, 1951

I offered my day for Father Campeau's undertakings but still find it very difficult to pray so probably gained very few merits. Received another lovely letter from Harold and he sent me over some goodies. Then he came to the window to inquire about me so I am not being neglected. I still miss my walks with him.

Saturday, April 14th, 1951

Three girls from on the front balcony sneaked out this evening and luckily for them they weren't caught. They went out the window and climbed down a rope and blanket that were tied together. We told them that it was a stupid thing to do but they will probably do it again. However, they are all very likeable girls although a bit too adventuresome at times.

Monday, April 16th, 1951

Today is six years that Harold has been a patient here in the Sanatorium.

Wednesday, April 18th, 1951

Father Campeau came for Confession and Communion and was surprised to learn that I had haemorrhaged and was back in bed. After Father's little talk and receiving Holy Communion, I am now feeling quite a bit better. We are very fortunate to have Father Campeau.

Friday, April 20th, 1951

Received a letter from Harold this morning and saw him in person this afternoon. Harold received his discharge today so was within his legal rights to come up to visit me. This was a happy time for both of us. And now I hope with all my heart that Harold will keep well and never have to return to the Sanatorium.

Sunday, April 22nd, 1951

Mary and Nick came this afternoon and I had the pleasure of seeing Nick in his Air Force uniform for the first time. The teenage girls here think that "Nick looks so cute" and there seemed to be one of them peeking around every corner today as they all wanted to get a better look at him in uniform.

Sunday, April 29th, 1951

Harold came and we had a wonderful visit. He thinks that I am looking well again. I am happy.

Monday, May 7th, 1951

Dr. Carmichael said that my x-ray doesn't look any worse in spite of the haemorrhages that I had so I can go downstairs to the dining room for supper again. That is something to be very thankful for. However, I did have a big setback and won't be going home this month as was previously planned.

Sunday, May 20th, 1951

Ten years ago today I went back on the cure. Ten years ago today I walked out of the classroom for the last time. And I played my last game of baseball ten years ago today. Happy Anniversary Clara!

Harold came to see me today so it was a wonderful day. His visits bring the greatest joy possible.

Wednesday, May 23rd, 1951

George brought me a good pair of scissors and I am really pleased as the ones I had were practically useless.

A second six-year old meningitis victim came into room nine, next door to us and her name is Janet. Donna is very ill and was alone for a few days so I would go in every evening and read to her and help her with her night prayers.

Donna has a beautiful voice and makes good use of it in spite of being so ill as to be lying there almost death-like with eyes closed most of the day. We can hear her singing from in our room and to listen to her rendition of 'Mockingbird Hill' is a profoundly touching experience. I know that I will always think of Donna anytime that I will hear this song for as long as I shall live.

Saturday, May 26th, 1951

I still go in every evening to visit my two dear sweet little friends next door. Janet wants to make her First Communion and she is learning her Catechism and prayers very quickly. She is such a bright little girl. Donna had already made her First Communion when she came into the hospital.

Friday, June 1st, 1951

Father Campeau brought us Communion and I offered mine for Father's intentions and hope that I was able to help him in some small way.

Phyllis went home for good and we are going to miss her very much. Phyllis is a great person and a good friend and we all wish the best for her.

Donna and Janet still enjoy our evening sessions and when I'm not there on the stroke of seven they start yelling for me to go to them.

Wednesday, June 6th, 1951

Dr. Carmichael called several of us into the room to be fluoroscoped and he let us see ourselves and each other on the screen. My left side looks weird where the seven ribs are removed. The right side isn't as bad as there are only four ribs removed.

After we were through, Dr. Carmichael remarked "Clara is the only thoracoplasty patient here in the Sanatorium with enough sense not to be carrying on with a love affair." That remark caused considerable but quiet chuckling among the other patients.

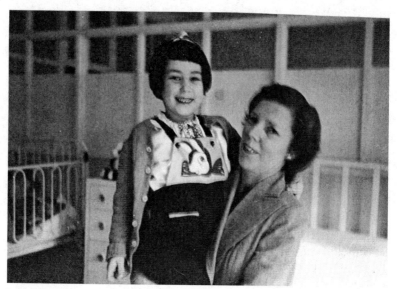

Royal Ottawa San – Janet and her mother.

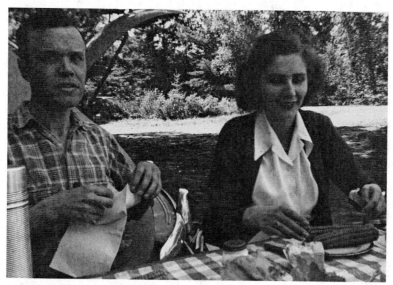

June 25, 1951. A Wonderful Day.
Clara Raina and Harold Mouré at Lac Philippe.

Dr. Carmichael has seen Harold and me together so often but just doesn't suspect anything and as a rule he is extremely wise. On the other hand, he sure perks up if he just sees me speaking with another man, even once. Maybe Dr. Carmichael feels that Harold is protecting me and actually he would be right.

Saturday, June 9th, 1951

I had the stomach flu so didn't go downstairs for my meals today and the nurses said that Janet and Donna were very concerned when I failed to pass by their door at mealtime. They wanted to know if I would be well enough to read to them this evening. Seven p.m. – Donna, Janet and I had our usual session and I was thrilled to see such happy little girls. They are wonderful for the morale.

Monday, June 25th, 1951

Dr. Carmichael let me have the day out to go on a picnic to Lac Philippe with some friends. Ralph, Harold and this other girl are all home now and I am the only one left in the Sanatorium and I had to be back here for 9:30 p.m. as usual. Another wonderful, wonderful day.

Wednesday, July 18th, 1951

This morning I put candles on a table in Janet's room in preparation for her First Communion. Then Velma and I received Holy Communion in the room with Janet and Donna and Janet looked like a little angel after receiving Communion from Father Campeau.

This evening Janet, Donna and I said our beads together before I read them their stories. I can't help but love these little girls – they are so different and very interesting, each in her own way. Janet has very dark hair and Donna is so blond.

Saturday, July 28th, 1951

Dad went home today and we are all concerned as he has not made any progress but, on the contrary, he seems to be getting worse. Ralph and Lou came for Dad and the four of us had a good visit together.

Louis looks nice in his Air Force uniform, and I am becoming a very popular girl because I have so many eligible brothers.

Sunday, July 29th, 1951

Harold came and we had a lovely visit out on the lawn. We made a bargain. Harold will pray for Dad and I will pray for his aunt.

Sunday, August 5th, 1951

Harold came and I was very surprised to see him again – he comes so often. I honestly feel that it would be impossible for Heaven to contain greater happiness than what I experience whenever I am with Harold and this thought really frightens me. If I have already reached the peak capacity for human happiness by just being with Harold, then the thought of marriage and even greater happiness would be impossible to obtain. Something would have to happen. The closest comparison that I can make, I think, would be to take a balloon and blow it to full capacity until one more breath would cause it to burst. I am filled to capacity with happiness when I am with Harold. More air will burst the balloon. More happiness would cause me to burst and I would disintegrate. For this reason there are times that I try searching for flaws in Harold so I won't like him as much as I do but it's no use as I never can find any faults. I always come to the same conclusion. Harold is just perfect and I love him very much.

Tuesday, September 4th, 1951
(during my two weeks at home)

Harold came out from Ottawa and will spend a couple of days at our place.

After lunch Ralph, Harold, another girl and I left for an outing and our first stop was a visit to Fort Wellington in Prescott. We looked at all the displays inside the Fort and signed our names in the visitors' book and then we went on to catch the ferry and crossed over to Ogdensburg, New York. Upon our arrival in the States we walked around and window shopped for a while and then we entered a Cocktail Lounge and ordered a drink.

I explained to Harold that this was my first cocktail ever and that I did not understand anything about the nature of drinking. But I knew that I did not wish to become intoxicated and would trust him to see to it that my wishes were carried out.

We each had one drink and then we went to see a movie. We sat in the back row and there were no solid walls behind us but it was more like Venetian blinds. Harold was in a very comical mood and he proceeded to close all the slats in the blinds that were directly behind us and while performing his task he remarked "We just can't have people standing there peeking in at us during the movie." Maybe the one cocktail that each of us had was a powerful one but we were all in a jovial mood by now and Ralph almost convinced Harold to offer some popcorn to the two very sedate ladies that were seated on the other side of him.

The movie starred Bing Crosby in *Here Comes The Groom* and we thoroughly enjoyed the show.

After we left the theatre we went back to have one more cocktail each and then things became even more humorous than before. Harold and Ralph tried harder than ever to convince me that I was drunk. And Harold held my arm all the way to the car and he said that I needed his help to remain on my feet in the condition that I was in. Then when we got down to the dock the men tried to convince us girls that we had missed the last ferry back and would have to remain in the States overnight. Just as I was beginning to have a few doubts the ferry came along and we were soon back in Canada again.

We stopped off in Prescott and had a bite to eat and then we came home. I am as happy as can be. It was such a wonderful day.

Wednesday, September 5th, 1951

After breakfast Harold and I went for a long walk, just like old times. Later on the four of us walked across the road and then we sat down in the sand pile and chatted for a while. Before leaving for Ottawa, Harold invited me to go to his place on Saturday.

Saturday, September 8th, 1951

I got up bright and early and prepared for the big day ahead. My two weeks at home were over and it was time to say goodbye to the family again.

Ralph dropped me off at Mourés and then he went to the Sanatorium for his pneumothorax treatment. Harold took me to the Archives this morning and I found it very interesting as I had never been there before. When we were through at the Archives we rendez-voused with Ralph and George and then the four of us went to see *Captain Hornblower* at the Capital Theatre. After the movie we returned to Mourés for supper and we all enjoyed the food and the visiting.

Another wonderful day was drawing to a close and it was time to return to the Sanatorium once more.

Sunday, September 9th, 1951

Harold came to see me this afternoon and as usual it was so good so see him. Jerry and Marion also dropped in and it was nice to see them too.

Wednesday, September 12th, 1951

Doctor Carmichael put me up on exercise again but I am only to go out when the weather is favourable.

Saturday, October 6th, 1951

The girls made a birthday party for me and Miss W., our night nurse, also had a gift for me. It is a red neckband with a clip and I was instructed to wear it the next time that Harold comes to see me. She is still doing her utmost to get Harold and I married to each other. She is a real eager beaver if ever I saw one. That's our Miss W. – the matchmaker.

Wednesday, October 10th, 1951

Both little girls next door were progressing nicely and then Donna had a serious relapse and is now in a semi-coma. However, Janet continues to improve and is very bright and alert.

Sunday, October 14th, 1951

When Harold came to visit me today the Eager Beaver cornered him for a long chat and she made one final attempt to convince him that he and I should eventually get married. She is so certain that we were made for each other and that we would be ecstatically happy together. This is Miss W.'s last day here as she is returning to England. Miss Clement overheard Miss

W. speaking with Harold and was highly amused when she later repeated the conversation to me.

Friday, October 19th, 1951

Harold was in for a checkup and the doctor gave him permission to return to work but they are still somewhat concerned over his left lung so he is to take it easy over the weekends and rest as much as possible. Harold said he won't be able to come as often to see me now but that he will write instead. I am so happy for him and will pray hard so that he will keep well.

Little Donna underwent surgery at the Civic Hospital and returned today with her head bandaged. She is extremely ill and there is very little hope for her recovery.

Saturday, November 3rd, 1951

Ralph came for his pneumothorax treatment and Mother sent along a whole roasted chicken and needless to say Velma, Denise and I sure enjoyed the treat.

Tuesday, November 6th, 1951

Received a letter from Harold and he is very happy to be back at work but misses his visits here. I miss him too but would much rather have him resting instead of coming here and overdoing himself. Harold returned to his former place of employment where he used to do the bookkeeping nearly seven years ago.

Saturday, November 17th, 1951

Mayor Charlotte Whitton was supposed to come to the Preventorium this afternoon to promote the sale of the TB Christmas Seals.[24] The photographer and the other men wandered around speaking with the patients as they waited for Charlotte to put in an appearance and the photographer took a picture of Velma, Denise and me. Charlotte never did turn up and as the men prepared to leave one of them remarked, "just like a woman, they can never be trusted."

Monday, November 26th, 1951

I received a six page letter from Harold and I am getting very lonesome for him but know he has to rest. However, we do write to each other frequently.

Friday, November 30th, 1951

I bought a cute little hat from out of the catalogue and it only cost a dollar and ninety-eight cents. It is brown and green velvet and is the first new hat that I have bought in years.

Saturday, December 8th, 1951

Jean, an old roommate of mine, is in the Civic Hospital having foot surgery and Dr. Carmichael told me to go and visit her while on my exercise this afternoon.

Denise came along with me and after we saw Jean we went to visit Miss Rogers, one of our nurses, who is also a patient in the Civic Hospital.

---

24 "Charlotte Whitton was the first female mayor of a major city in Canada, but not the first female mayor in Canada. She served from 1951 to 1956 and again from 1960 to 1964." http://en.wikipedia.org/wiki/Charlotte_Whitton; 10/06/2010.

Saturday, December 15th, 1951

The Legion of Mary put on a Christmas Party for the patients this afternoon and there was lots to eat and presents for everyone. Father Campeau and another priest attended the party and they took several pictures. A good time was had by all.

Saturday, December 23rd, 1951

I was given five days of leave for Christmas and am spending the first two days in Ottawa with Mary. Harold came over today and I was so happy to see him again but there was also a feeling of sadness and concern as I do not think that he looks well. Harold has a cold and seems so frail. This means that I will have to pray harder than ever.

Harold gave me two Christmas presents. One gift is a little unusual but is a gift that I will treasure for the rest of my life. It is a book Harold had as a child and there was a note enclosed saying he hopes that I will keep this book for myself. As I delve into this delightful story I feel as though Harold is sharing his childhood with me and I am overwhelmed with happiness. Harold must really understand what I am like to know that this gift would be so pleasing to me.

Monday, December 24th, 1951

Mary and I got up bright and early and went to confession and seven o'clock Mass at St. Patrick's Church. Then a little later Mary, her boyfriend, and I took the bus home to Kemptville. I got car sick so the bus driver stopped at North Gower and bought me a bromoseltzer. He was a very considerate man and I really appreciated his kindness.

Wednesday, December 26th, 1951

We are all concerned over Dad's health as he has lost over twenty pounds since coming home from the hospital. Otherwise, we all had a nice festive season.

Before returning to the Sanatorium this evening we went to Mourés for a couple of hours and Harold looks even worse than he did on Sunday. I am *very* concerned.

Monday, December 31st, 1951

Tomorrow will be New Year's Day and what I would like more than anything else is to be able to visit inside St. Francis' church on Wellington Street. I want to thank God for the favours received during the past year and to ask for the courage that will be needed to face the coming year. Somehow I feel a great need for God's assistance and there are so many things to pray for.

I was going to make some New Year resolutions but may not keep them for long so decided that I would write a prayer instead and I will say it every day during 1952. I know that it is poorly composed but God will understand what I mean.

"Dear Sacred Heart of Jesus and Blessed Virgin Mary, please help me to make 1952 the best year of my life and the most pleasing to Thee. Help me to be kind and patient to all those around me and bless everyone who has helped me in any way.

Please watch over my family's health and all the patients in the Sanatorium and give them the courage to accept their crosses. If it is your Holy will, please restore Harold and me to good health and grant us much happiness together and help us to ever be your loving children.

Please take special care of my dear parents, brothers and sisters, Father Campeau, Doctor Carmichael, Miss Clement, also all other priests, doctors and nurses. Watch over all our service men and grant eternal rest to all the souls in purgatory. If any of us should die during the coming year be with us at the last hour and help us to die a holy death. I beg of Thee for these favours if it be for the good of our souls. Amen."

CHAPTER TWENTY-ONE

A YEAR TO REMEMBER

January 1, 1952 – October 16, 1952
Twenty-Five Years, Three Months – Twenty-Six Years

Tuesday, January 1ˢᵗ, 1952

This morning Doctors Carmichael and Kubilius made rounds to wish us all a Happy New Year.

Then this afternoon my wish was granted. A kind friend drove me to make a visit in St. Francis Church on Wellington Street and I had an opportunity to say some special prayers. This was a great comfort for me as I have some very uneasy feelings as to what the New Year might have in store for us.

Tuesday, January 8ᵗʰ, 1952

I haven't heard from Harold since Christmas and am very worried.

Sunday, January 13ᵗʰ, 1952

Ralph, Lou, George and Nick came this afternoon and it was so nice seeing all of them. Ralph said that he ran into Jerry and was told that Harold is quite ill at home. I am very concerned.

Tuesday, January 15th, 1952

I received a letter from Harold and he has been very ill. He had severe nosebleeds and had to have his nose packed. Needless to say, my worries continue.

Saturday, January 19th, 1952

Dr. Carmichael has new false teeth.

Thursday, January 24th, 1952

I received another letter from Harold and things do not sound good. He is still running a temperature.

Lou is stationed at Winnipeg Air Base and takes off for there today.

Friday, January 25th, 1952

I received a letter from Father Patrick Peyton thanking me for my Christmas card and letter.

Saturday, February 2nd, 1952

Harold was admitted to the Whitney Building and was transfused with three pints of blood. When I heard the bad news I shed many tears.

Sunday, February 3rd, 1952

The orderly from the Whitney came over to give me a letter from Harold and I was so pleased to hear from him. He said that he is only supposed to be here for a few days – just to receive transfusions.

Denise was discharged today and we are going to miss her but it is always nice to see a patient going home. So many aren't walking when they leave, so we all rejoice when we can verbally bid them adieu.

Wednesday, February 6th, 1952

King George the Sixth died early today.

Friday, February 8th, 1952

I managed to get up into the Whitney Building to visit Harold for a while this afternoon and we were so happy to see each other again. We have rarely broken any of the rules around here but I broke the rules today by going to visit Harold without having the doctor's permission. Even though we do have tuberculosis we are still human beings and may enjoy seeing each other, but San Romances are a 'no no' around here.

Harold has had numerous blood tests and a Dr. Fisher came to take a marrow test from his breastbone. I am very concerned as I fear that there is something seriously wrong with Harold.

I am knitting a sleeveless blue sweater for Harold and I hope that he will be able to wear it.

Saturday, February 9th, 1952

Ralph and Nick came today after visiting with Harold. He had just finished writing a five page letter to me so asked Ralph to bring it along over with him. Harold mentions that he likes the little hat that I wore yesterday. That was my $1.98 hat that I got from catalogue shopping.

Sunday, February 10th, 1952

We attended Mass at the Whitney this morning and Harold sent down a letter for me with one of the other patients. I met Mrs. Mouré while out walking this afternoon and I feel very sorry for her because of Harold's illness again.

Saturday, February 16th, 1952

Harold and I write to each other every day and in today's letter he tells me that he is going to be transferred to the Civic Hospital on Monday. He still gets transfusions but the doctors aren't really telling him anything and keep avoiding his questions. After asking some of the nurses various medical questions we are beginning to suspect that Harold has leukemia. I am not happy with the results of our detective work.

We are all praying hard for Harold and are saying several different novenas for him. The Protestants as well as the Catholics are taking part in these prayers.

Sunday, February 17th, 1952

I had the doctor's permission to visit another patient at the Whitney but spent forty-five minutes with Harold. I wish that we could legally visit with each other as I do love him so much.

Wednesday, February 20th, 1952

Harold's letters continue to arrive daily and he is very pleased that I am knitting a sweater for him. However, his letters indicate that he is somewhat downhearted since his arrival at the Civic Hospital as the doctors still aren't telling him what the matter is with him.

One of our favourite nurses who works both here at the Sanatorium and at the Civic came to see me this afternoon as she felt that I was entitled to the information that she gave me. She has learned the results of Harold's tests and it is almost certain that he has leukemia. Even though I already suspected leukemia I was still hoping that it wasn't so. The tears flowed for hours this evening until the nurse finally brought me a sleeping pill and said she figured that I could use it.

I am just hoping that no one will tell the doctors nor some of the nurses about Harold and me as I am planning to sneak over to the Civic to see him when I go on exercise. The ones who disapprove of San Romances will keep a very close watch over me if they become suspicious. Harold has told me not to sneak over as he knows I would be in serious trouble if caught.

Saturday, February 23rd, 1952

At first Harold advised me against sneaking over but in the letter today he says that he would very much like to see me if I can manage a way to get there without being caught. Harold and I have never liked nor have we believed in breaking the rules but there are times when we have to make decisions and be prepared to suffer the consequences. And I believe that the time has now come for me to take advantage of the first opportunity that presents itself for me to go and see him.

Sunday, February 24th, 1952

Father Campeau said Mass for us and later we spoke about Harold. Father said that Harold is one of the nicest men that he knows.

This afternoon I ventured over to visit Harold and we were very happy to see each other. Harold was receiving another transfusion and my heart ached for him. The doctors still aren't telling him anything and I really think that he is the type of person who should be told the truth. I can't tell Harold he has leukemia as the nurse who told me would then be involved. However I am very grateful to this nurse for telling me the truth.

Monday, February 25th, 1952

Another wonderful letter from Harold and he doesn't want me to worry over him.

I had told Harold about all the prayers and novenas being said for him by all the patients here at the Preventorium. To this he commented that he is very fortunate and appreciates all the prayers but feels that he is receiving more than his share and hopes that we won't mind but that he has asked Our Lord to apply a portion of our prayers to other less fortunate patients in the Civic and to the ones who are in great pain. When I first read these words I really felt defeated and wanted to shout, "No Lord, you can't do that and I do mind. All the prayers that I say for Harold, I want them applied to him and to no one else." Then after meditating for a few moments I resigned myself to Harold's wishes and if it were possible my love for him would have increased even more. Harold is a very kind and generous person and I have never heard him criticize others nor have I ever heard anyone criticize Harold.

My heart continues to break but I must hold back the tears until after the lights are out at night as there are too many people who must not know about us or my visits to the Civic would come to an abrupt end. It can be very difficult to go around laughing and smiling when my heart is breaking inside. I wish that I was away from the Sanatorium so that I could visit Harold whenever I want to.

Tuesday, February 26th, 1952

Phyllis came in their car and she drove me to see Harold and then she brought me back again. Phyllis is a great person and a good friend so Harold was very pleased to see both of us. Harold was receiving more transfusions but in spite of it he was very cheerful.

Thursday, February 28th, 1952

I sneaked over to the Civic again today and I took Harold the blue sweater that I knit for him. As usual we were so pleased to see each other.

Sunday, March 2nd, 1952

Dad took a bad turn and was anointed today but he is going to remain at home and Mother and Ralph will care for him. Now both Dad and Harold are very ill.

Tuesday, March 4th, 1952

Ralph came at noon to take me home as Dad is seriously ill. I wish this illness would not all come at once as I did not like leaving Ottawa while Harold is so ill. However, we are very thankful for the way that Dad is accepting his illness. His spirits are good.

Wednesday, March 5th, 1952

Mary and George came home today and we sent telegrams to Nick and Lou asking them to come home too.

Dad took another bad turn and Father Quinn came and recited the prayers for the dying. Dad continues to be very brave so it makes things much easier for Mother and the rest of the family.

Friday, March 7th, 1952

Nick arrived and then Lou flew in from Winnipeg and when Dad saw all of his children he shed tears of joy.

Saturday, March 8th, 1952

Ralph brought me back to the San today and I felt very sad when I had to leave Dad. This is an extremely difficult time. I was thankful to be at home with Father but with Harold so ill too I wanted to be in Ottawa so I could go and see him. What I really wanted was to be both places at the same time.

Sunday, March 9th, 1952

There was Mass at the Whitney this morning and Father Campeau asked the patients to pray for Dad.

I went to see Harold this afternoon and we had a whole hour alone and it was wonderful. The doctor told him that his latest blood test was three times better than the previous one was and we are both very excited. If only God will cure him. I am still saying so many prayers for both Dad and Harold, even if Harold is sharing his prayers.

Tuesday, March 11th, 1952

I went to see Harold and we had another wonderful visit. His cousin Doris was also there visiting with him.

Wednesday, March 12th, 1952

This is 'movie night' but I didn't have any desire to go as I can only think of Dad and Harold. I stayed in bed and prayed instead. I asked God to give Dad and Harold the courage that they need at this critical time.

Thursday, March 13th, 1952

I had planned to visit Harold today but the nurse in charge may have heard rumours as she told us to check with her before leaving on exercise and then to check in upon our return. Officially I am on fifteen minutes exercise so there was no way that I could walk so many blocks in that time so I was defeated. And I am heartbroken. Then to make matters even worse there was no letter from Harold today.

Friday, March 14th, 1952

Another day without the opportunity to see Harold and another day without a letter.

How much longer will I be able to carry on this charade pretending that all is well when my heart is breaking inside?

An already difficult day reached a climax at about nine this evening. Miss Rogers, the night nurse, brought me news of Harold. He is much worse and wishes to see me. Now that the cat is out of the bag I hope the doctor won't prevent me from going to the Civic tomorrow as I must see Harold.

Saturday, March 15th, 1952

Miss Clement brought me another message this morning and it also states that Harold wishes to see me. He was anointed on Thursday and has been given about one week to live. I am heartbroken and hope that no one will try to prevent me from going to the Civic Hospital this afternoon. Miss Clement has known all along about Harold and me and she is a good friend. She says nothing and I have been assured that she will not interfere as long as I do not involve her.

Now that my secret is out I inquired from a nurse as to what unfavourable remarks Dr. Carmichael had made. At first she denied that anything was said but once I convinced her that I have been in the Sanatorium long enough to know differently she reluctantly told me the truth. At first Dr. Carmichael was very hurt and upset as he remarked, "I just cannot understand how Clara could have a San Romance for so long without anyone telling me about it." He was very hurt as he felt that he had a right to this information (he saw us together often enough but it never sank in).

The nurse said that once Dr. Carmichael had finally digested the shocking news he became quite concerned regarding my health. He said that if Harold is more than a casual friend his death will be very hard on me. And that means I will have to endure two deaths in the near future as both Harold and Dad's deaths are imminent.

Dr. Carmichael issued permission for me to go and see Harold this afternoon but he is quite unhappy with this latest bit of startling news.

When I arrived at Harold's bedside he had another visitor and he introduced us to each other and then this other girl left shortly afterwards. Harold then told me about the promise that she has made if he recovers and he appreciates this gesture of hers.

Harold looked very poorly and it was obvious from the start that he was much worse than the last time that I had seen him. Suddenly I noticed that Harold had difficulty breathing so I decided to go and ask the nurse for another pillow even though Harold insisted that he was alright and told me not to worry. I put the extra pillow underneath his head but that didn't help and he began to perspire profusely and still insisted that he was fine. I knew differently and went for the nurse. Then the rush was on and Harold was hooked up to the oxygen as the medical staff worked over him. Just at this time Harold's cousin Doris, the nurse, walked in and I was so relieved to see a relative of his.

The medical staff was still working over Harold when it was time for me to return to the Sanatorium and I hated to leave. However, Doris came over to the Sanatorium later to tell me that Harold's condition was slightly improved since getting oxygen.

This has been one bad day and there may be worse ones ahead. I am determined that I will sneak over to the Civic tomorrow. A good nurse is going to be on duty here so it may not be too difficult, but I can't imagine what will happen by Monday. The doctors will see to it by then that I will be closely guarded!

Sunday, March 16th, 1952

I went to see Harold this afternoon and he is very ill and is in an oxygen tent. In spite of being so ill there was so much that he wanted to tell me and he even managed to smile that wonderful smile of his several times. I tried to smile too but my eyes were burning with tears that were waiting to be shed and my heart was breaking apart.

Harold told me that when the doctor was in this morning that he insisted that he be told about his illness. Then the doctor told him that he has leukemia. I never let on that I already knew, but I often thought that Harold is the type of person who should have been told the nature of his illness much sooner. Harold said that he would very much like to get better – but – then he shrugged his shoulders and there was a look of intense sorrow showing in his eyes. Then the sorrowful look was replaced with a big smile and even a sparkle in his eyes as he said "We did have many wonderful times together and you will have those memories." Harold told me that I am not to worry over him but to see to it that I get well. Speaking was very difficult but he wanted to talk as long as I stayed with him. Never before in my life was it this difficult to leave someone. Harold's facial expressions again changed a few times, from a smile to a look of extreme sorrow and I am sure that I must have looked the same way as I kept looking back at him and slowly walked out of the room.

Those were very sad but very precious moments that we shared together.

After I arrived back at the Preventorium many tears were shed and I still stormed Heaven for a miracle.

St. Patrick's Day, Monday, March 17th, 1952

Just as *Danny Boy* was being sung on the radio this morning Miss Clement came to inform me that Harold had died at around nine o'clock last night. This is the saddest thing that has ever happened to me in my whole life. Yet I am thankful to God for having allowed me to know this wonderful man and for all the happiness that we shared.

Everyone is being very kind and dear little Louise tried so hard to be extra sweet. First she made me a St. Patrick's Day card and then she gave me a chocolate bar. Then Louise went over to Babs and I overheard her whispering "Don't you think that I am being real nice to Clara? First I made the St. Patrick's Day card for her and now I gave her that chocolate bar and it is a big one and it cost twenty cents and it is my favourite kind of bar." Then Louise returned to ask me when I intended to eat the chocolate bar. "Right now, if you will help me eat it" I replied. Louise was pleased with this decision that I had made and she was a real help in my time of sorrow. Sometimes there can be a bit of comedy even in the greatest of tragedies.

Never before in my life have I ever felt God's presence as close as He was today.[25] As I lay there weeping it seemed as though God was standing by the left side of my bed and wanted me to know that He was even more sorrowful than I was. That He had heard all of my prayers and novenas but that there just

---

25 There have been many times throughout the years when God has seemed to be so far away and totally unaware of my existence. And how I longed for His closeness once again like I experienced on March 17th, 1952. God's entire attention seemed to be focused on me for a while that day and now I know how fortunate I was then even though I did not fully realize it at the time. It must be true that God never sends us more than we can bear without coming to our assistance even though this is hard to believe at times.

wasn't any alternative – that it was necessary for Harold to die and He wanted me to trust Him.

Tuesday, March 18th, 1952

Phyllis came this afternoon and took me to Harold's wake and I saw him for the last time. I hope that God will give me the courage to accept this great cross. The flowers I sent to Harold's wake were in the form of a cross and they looked nice. I also gave Father Campeau money to say a Mass for the repose of Harold's soul.

Wednesday, March 19th, 1952

Father Campeau brought us Communion and I prayed for Dad and for Harold. Harold's funeral was this morning and I wasn't able to go and am very sad today. When Dr. Carmichael gave me permission to go to Harold's wake he said that I would not be able to go to the funeral though as the strain might be too much for me as I will shortly have to face Dad's death too.

Thursday, March 20th, 1952

I received a letter from Mother and there were a few words at the bottom of the page that Dad had written in spite of being so ill.

I haven't been going for my walks as I just can't get in the mood for exercise.

Tuesday, March 25th, 1952

Dick Mouré and his girl friend Leanore Higgins came to visit me and I was so pleased to see both of them. Dick brought me a prayer book that Harold had willed to me.

Thursday, March 27th, 1952

I finally went back outside for my walk this afternoon as I have to pull myself together and carry on.

Sunday, March 30th, 1952

The Mass said here at the Preventorium this morning was offered for Harold and I think this was very kind of Father Campeau.

Saturday, April 12th, 1952

I have received several lovely Easter cards and some beautiful flowers among which were two pretty roses from Bert and Babs. My family and friends are so good to me.

Janet went home today and we are all so pleased that she recovered. She is one of the little girls who I used to read to. Unfortunately Donna passed away early in December but she will always be remembered for the way she sang Mockingbird Hill.

Thursday, April 17th, 1952

Dr. Carmichael ordered some tests for Maureen and me as they are planning to give us the new drug 'Rimifon' as soon as the necessary tests are completed. Rimifon is the latest drug out to combat tuberculosis and I hope that it will help us.

Sunday, April 20th, 1952

I was summoned to the desk after breakfast and for the second time in five weeks Miss Clement informed me of the death of a loved one. Ralph had phoned to say that Dad passed away peacefully at two o'clock this morning. Even though we feel badly we are still thankful for the way that Dad accepted his illness and imminent death so cheerfully.

Monday, April 21st, 1952

I was given a few days leave to be with the family as Dad is being waked at home in Kemptville. There were several people here for the wake this evening and I was especially pleased to see Dick Mouré and his girlfriend Leanore and Jerry and Marion Lachance.

There always seemed to be one or two members of the family crying and I suppose that I shed about an equal amount of tears. Only when I cried I was full of guilt as I was never sure if I was crying because of Dad or if my tears were still being shed for Harold. I would have liked more time to come to terms with myself over Harold's death before losing my Father. However we do not have a choice over these matters and it is so difficult when a person has to lose two loved ones so close together.

Wednesday, April 23rd, 1952

Dad's funeral was yesterday and I feel very sorry for Mother as she is going to be so lonesome and lost for a while.

Ralph drove Mary and me back to Ottawa this afternoon and Mother, Jimmy and Anne came along for the drive. When I returned to my room there was a lovely bouquet of flowers on my bedside table that the nurses had bought for me. Everyone has been wonderful these past several weeks.

Sunday, April 27th, 1952

Father Campeau said Mass here at the Preventorium this morning and he offered the Mass for Dad. This was very comforting to me.

Friday, May 2nd, 1952

Father Campeau brought us Communion and I offered my day for the success of his priestly undertakings.

Doctor Harper put the order in the book today for Maureen and me to start taking 'Rimifon', three pills daily. Then he discontinued my exercise as he feels that this drug might work better if I rest as much as possible. However, I can still go downstairs to the dining room for my meals. We were told to report any reactions that we may have from the drug.

Monday, May 5th, 1952

My breathing is really bothering me in an unusual and weird way and I wonder if the Rimifon could be causing this discomfort. I told Miss Clement about my breathing difficulties and Dr. Harper examined me.

Sunday, May 25th, 1952

We had Mass downstairs this morning and Father Campeau looked exhausted. We are worried over our priest and think that he should get more rest.

I have been so blue lately as this has been a very bad year with so much illness in our family. Then apart from these other problems there were the deaths of Dad and Harold. Last December I had a very uneasy feeling of what lay ahead in 1952 and now I can understand why.

Tuesday, May 27th, 1952

A new nurse was on this evening so some of the girls sneaked downstairs and went into the kitchen looking for food. All they could find was a gallon tin of tomato juice so they brought it back upstairs with them. Then we all got our fill of Vitamin C as we had to empty the can and destroy all the evidence of the great juice robbery.

Thursday, June 5th, 1952

Father Campeau came for Confession and he gave me a good little talk and I hope that it will help me to get over this blue mood that I am experiencing. Father always seems to know what to say to make people feel better afterwards. He is truly a good person and a good priest.

Saturday, June 14th, 1952

Ralph came for pneumo and brought along a roasted chicken that Mother had prepared for the girls in this room. Babs, Bert, Priscilla and I ate the chicken after 'lights out' this evening as we didn't want to eat it in front of the other patients who were wandering in and out of our room because there was just enough for the four of us to have a good feed. Delicious treat!

Friday, June 20th, 1952

Today is the Feast of the Sacred Heart so I read the Mass and said some other prayers.

This evening I re-read the letters that Harold had written to me and this made me feel very lonesome.

Tuesday, July 8th, 1952

George brought me some chop suey and I really enjoyed the treat.

Tuesday, July 22nd, 1952

I finished reading *The Confessions of St. Augustine* and found it a very impressive and interesting book.

Friday, July 25th, 1952

I lost six pounds since I started taking Rimifon and now weigh 113 pounds. My haemoglobin is down to 76% so Dr.

Harper ordered iron pills for me to take three times daily. My sedimentation is four.

Wednesday, July 30th, 1952

Mary was taken to the Civic Hospital and had her appendix removed. I sure hope that she is going to be alright.

Friday, August 1st, 1952

Father Campeau brought us Communion and he told me he has seen Mary in the Civic Hospital and that she is coming along nicely. I am so relieved and thankful.

Dr. Harper examined me and said that it doesn't seem as though Rimifon has been of any help to me so he will discontinue the medication. Then the doctor ordered a tonic that I will get three times daily as well as the iron pills that were prescribed last week.

Friday, August 22nd, 1952

This morning we were taken to the special Grandstand Performance given by the Ottawa Exhibition at Lansdowne Park. Our driver drove us around Uplands Airport and through Ottawa South and then he stopped at a store to buy us chocolate bars. He was a very kind man who is a diabetic so he could not eat any of the chocolate bars himself.

Occasionally I get car sick and this was one of my really bad days and I am supposed to leave tomorrow for two weeks of vacation at home. Just the thought of stepping inside a car again does not appeal to me at this time.

When we returned from the Exhibition there was a letter waiting for me from an ex-San patient. He says that he wants to see me and would like to come and visit me often. I do not want him to come at all. I do not want a consolation prize to replace Harold. And I am *not* going to answer his letter!

Saturday, August 23rd, 1952

Dr. Harper brought over some Gravol for me to take so I wouldn't get car sick on the way home.

Mother and Ralph came for me and Mother had packed a nice picnic lunch for us to eat on our way home. We sat along the Driveway and watched the sailboats out in the water as we ate our sandwiches and I enjoyed this outing before going home.

Monday, August 25th 1952

It is nice to be home and I have been playing a lot of cards with the family. Then Jim drove me down to the old place in Nick's car and he drives quite well. He is still too young to drive on the road.

Mother and I walked down to Chapmans' store this evening to buy some hamburgers and soft drinks. They make delicious hamburgers and sell a lot of them.

Tuesday, August 26th, 1952

Ralph took me to see a ball game in Kemptville this evening and then we went to visit Noni afterwards. Noni is the person who made Winganonimous, the little stuffed bear when she was a patient in the Sanatorium.

Wednesday, August 27th, 1952

It is a warm, ninety degrees so we ate our supper outside and then we stayed out and watched the stars late into the night.

The family is treating me very well but I miss Harold so much and can't help but think about the good times that we had last year when I was home for two weeks.

Wednesday, September 3rd, 1952

Kemptville voted to see if liquor can be sold but they lost out so it's still dry.

Saturday, September 6th, 1952

I felt lonely when I had to return to the San today but am thankful for the past two weeks that I had at home with my family in Kemptville.

Monday, September 15th, 1952

The only radio program that we are allowed to listen to after lights out at night is *Lux Theatre* that is on every Monday night from nine to ten p.m. *Here Comes The Groom* was on this evening and it brought back many memories as this was the movie that we saw with Harold in Ogdensburg, New York, last year. Tomorrow will be six months since Harold died and I still do a lot of crying after lights are out at night.

Friday, September 26th, 1952

I have a sore swollen nose and when Dr. Harper was walking into our room to examine me the girls on the balcony loudly sang "Rudolph The Red Nosed Reindeer!" The doctor ordered penicillin for me and the other patients never left poor Rudolph alone.

Tuesday, September 30th, 1952

Dr. Harper examined my nose and said that he won't have to cut it off after all. I have had to take a lot of teasing over this nose infection. First it was the patients and now it is the doctor. However, I do agree that Rudolph and I would have made a great team.

Sunday, October 5th, 1952

The leaves are changing colour and are very beautiful so I spend a lot of time just lying here in my bed and looking at the big tree outside my window.

Wednesday, October 8th, 1952

Dr. Carmichael said that he looked through my chart this morning as they are planning to send me home soon unless they decide on some other form of treatment to give me.

Monday, October 13th, 1952

There was no Thanksgiving leave given this year but we were served a delicious turkey dinner which helped to ease our disappointment.

Mrs. Amon returned from her holidays and she brought us each a drinking glass as a souvenir of her trip. She is always a pleasant nurse to have around and is well liked by all the patients.

Thursday, October 16th, 1952

Even though moisture can still be heard on my left lung the doctors are going to allow me to go home after I have a Broncoscopy examination.

CHAPTER TWENTY-TWO

SANDWICH A-LA-MOUSE

Saturday, October 18, 1952
Twenty-Six Years

Saturday, October 18th, 1952

When we were outside after supper we found a dead mouse on the window sill and the sight of it activated a few brain cells and then we swung into action. The mouse was cautiously wrapped in Kleenex tissue and carried inside. After that, one of the girls went to the kitchen and asked for two slices of buttered bread and moments later the mouse sandwich was nicely wrapped and ready to go. But first we had to decide who was the most worthy person to receive this gourmet treat and after concentrating for a few moments the decision was unanimous. The recipient would be a certain gentleman over at the Whitney Building. This fellow always teases us girls whenever he sees us and he uses the foulest language of anyone here in the Sanatorium. Minutes later one of our good natured nurses delivered the sandwich over to the Whitney Building.

Later on this evening as some of the men at the Whitney were sitting on their window sill in the balcony and some of the girls were doing likewise over here, we were wondering if there would be an exchange of words between the two buildings as we had all agreed to remain mum concerning the mouse. However, one of the girls surprised us when all of a sudden she yelled over and asked this fellow if he had had a good supper. Then there was a sudden eruption and the air almost turned blue between the two buildings. Actually this was one time that we couldn't blame the fellow for being angry, but he sure did use some foul language as he let off steam. And the other men wouldn't tell us either if the mouse sandwich did get bitten into or not. I think that I shall always check the contents of a sandwich from now on before I dare to bite into it.

CHAPTER TWENTY-THREE

LEAVING 'THE SAN' – EXCITEMENT AND APPREHENSION

Wednesday, October 29, 1952 – August 24, 1955
Twenty-Six Years – Twenty-Eight Years, Ten Months

Wednesday, October 29th, 1952

I was moved over to the Perley Building yesterday in order to have a broncoscopy examination at the Whitney Building at nine o'clock this morning. Dr. Harper told me that he did not find anything that will prevent me from going home.

Thursday, October 30th, 1952

The tests that were taken from my bronchial tubes are negative and I was brought back to the Preventorium this morning.

Dr. Harper has sent out some papers concerning my discharge that is to take place very shortly.

Friday, November 7th, 1952

Father Campeau came for Confession and Communion this morning and now I may not be seeing Father for quite a while as I am going home tomorrow.

I am excited about going home but am also quite apprehensive as it isn't as though I was well and able to participate in normal activities but I will have to remain on the cure at home and once again feel like a fish out of water. Those are not happy thoughts.

Miss Clement gave me a nice silk kerchief as a souvenir and she told me to let them know if ever I don't feel well and they will prepare a bed for my return. Dr. Carmichael came over to say goodbye and he told me to have a nice holiday.

The girls have been playing tricks on me all day. And every time I leave the room they either sew my sheets together or make a French bed so there is always a lot of work involved before I can get back into bed again. Then there are other problems as well – the girls won't allow me to do my own packing. They take over forcefully using the pretence that I look so tired. I would rather do my own packing so I will know where everything is when I arrive home but these girls are all good friends and I don't want to hurt their feelings.

Saturday, November 8th, 1952

Most of the doctors and several of the nurses have been in to wish me luck and to say goodbye. Dr. Harper said he hopes that I will surprise all of them and never have to return as a patient but only come back as a visitor to see them. He is a very nice doctor.

Ralph and Mary came to take me home and there were so many boxes. Either the girls are very poor packers or else I have more junk than I realized.

Sunday, November 9th, 1952

I was very tired when I arrived home yesterday so decided to wait until this morning to unpack and then do it while the family was at Mass.

The first box was nicely packed and contained part of my belongings but when I opened the second box I almost went into a state of shock and I knew why my friends insisted on doing the packing for me. Box Number Two held one bedpan filled with toilet paper and a note that said, "We don't want you to be lonesome so are sending some memories home with you." After recovering from the initial shock I began to laugh to myself and continued to chuckle until the family returned home from church. I could just vision the nurses in conference trying to figure out where on earth their bedpan had disappeared to. Then I wondered how I could secretly return the bedpan to the Sanatorium when I spotted the large suitcase that one of the kind packers had used so decided to return the bedpan inside her suitcase when it was taken back to her.

When I resumed the task of unpacking many more things were found that would have to be returned to the hospital and I continued to chuckle. If the girls failed as good packers they certainly succeeded in giving me many memories to remember them by.

Friday, December 12th, 1952

Nick is home on leave as he will soon be going to Germany. He seems to be forever treating us to Chapmans' good hamburgers. Chapmans is a restaurant and gas station that recently opened up just down the highway from us.

I made a bunting bag for Anne's doll and she is delighted with it.

Jim continues to be a lovable tease and I don't know what we would do without him around to liven things up.

Saturday, December 13th, 1952

Miss Clement phoned long distance for a chat and I was so pleased to hear from her as I still get very lonesome for the nurses and my friends back in the Sanatorium.

Monday, December 22nd, 1952

The Christmas cards are arriving in great numbers and it is always nice hearing from our friends. There was a letter from Father Campeau today and it brought with it a great deal of happiness for me.

Nick arrived home for five days of leave and everyone is happy that he will be home for Christmas. We are going to miss him when he goes to Germany.

Thursday, December 25th, 1952

We went to Midnight Mass last evening and everyone was up early again this morning. Mother prepared a delicious dinner for us but this was a very lonesome Christmas. I suppose one can easily understand why, as both Dad and Harold are missing this year.

Wednesday, December 31st, 1952

Once again I wrote a prayer for the New Year and I plan on saying it every day next year.

Monday, March 9th, 1953

Ralph opened a clothing store in the Finnerty Block in Kemptville and I hope that he will be very successful. Previously Ralph sold clothing from out of the garage at home and by going from door to door selling from his car.

Sunday, Monday, Tuesday (May 10th, 11th and 12th, 1953)

We took part in all of the Forty Hour Services that were held in the Holy Cross Church in Kemptville and I really enjoyed the sermons. I think the speaker's name was Father Carley.

Wednesday, August 19th, 1953

I was in Ottawa to have my eyes examined by Dr. Patterson and I will have to wear glasses all the time now. The eye examination cost seven dollars and my new glasses cost seventeen dollars.

Saturday, September 19th, 1953

I was in Ottawa so I went to see Mrs. Mouré and we had a nice visit. Then I went to St. Margaret Mary's Church and said a few prayers as this is the church that Harold used to belong to.

Saturday, December 5th, 1953

I had an appointment with Dr. Carmichael this morning to discuss the plainograph x-rays that were taken a week ago. I was told that the x-rays showed that there is still a cavity in the upper lobe of my left lung in spite of the thoracoplasty surgery so the doctors discussed the possibility of performing a lobectomy but decided that the risk would be too great.

Dr. Carmichael said that he doesn't want to make me feel badly but that I will have to be classified as being totally and permanently disabled. I am disappointed with the results but will try to make the best of it. There really isn't any other choice.

Dr. Carmichael gave me a large bottle of vitamin pills to bring home with me.

Thursday, December 17th, 1953

A lady came with a form for me to fill in so that I can receive a Disability Pension.

Saturday, January 30th, 1954

My heart has felt weird many times during the past few months and my ankles swell so I went to see Dr. Carmichael today and this is the first time I have told anyone about these symptoms. Dr. Carmichael said that my heart skips beats and he gave me some pills to take at bedtime. I asked Dr. Carmichael if this is serious and he said he doesn't think so but he wants to see me again in two weeks. I had one weird spell that I didn't tell the doctor about. I nearly keeled over and my mind went dull etc. and since then my sense of balance is bad. I'm always afraid of stumbling and my legs feel as though they might buckle from underneath me.

Saturday, February 13th, 1954

I was in to see Dr. Carmichael and he took some tests. He said that my circulation is bad and he gave me some more pills.

Thursday, February 18th, 1954

My first Disabled Person's Allowance cheque came today and it is for the sum of forty dollars. I will receive this amount every month from now on.

Saturday, May 17th, 1954

Ralph is very happy this evening as the sales in his store totalled $212.00 and this is the most that he has ever sold in one day.

Tuesday, May 25th, 1954

I entered the Whitney Building at the Royal Ottawa Sanatorium today as Dr. Carmichael wants to have me in here for two weeks for various heart tests and find out more about my swollen ankles.

I had x-rays and an electrocardiogram and this was my first cardiogram ever. Some Sanatoriums give electrocardiograms before they perform thoracoplasty surgery but the Royal Ottawa Sanatorium doesn't do it. At least I never had one taken before any of my surgeries. I was always told that my heart was good – until now.

Friday, June 4th, 1954

My sedimentation rate is four and all of my sputum tests are negative. Now Dr. Carmichael is supposed to get in touch with a heart specialist to discuss my electrocardiogram. The doctors have me going outside for walks twice daily. They check my pulse and swollen ankles before I leave and then when I return I report to Dr. Kubilius' office to have my pulse and ankles checked again.

I still haven't told the doctors about the one weird spell that I had one evening at home a while ago. I nearly passed out and I lost my balance and my mind was a little muddled for a while. It was as though I was robbed of a bit of my mentality and I couldn't concentrate as deeply as I could before this happened. I would like to discuss this with one of the doctors or with someone as I would like to be able to understand what really did happen to me. It was such a frightening experience and my sense of balance isn't back to normal yet, especially when I am tired. And then I worry that my legs will give away from underneath me and I will fall flat on my face.

Tuesday, June 8th, 1954

Yesterday I asked the doctor what is wrong with my heart and he replied, "Please don't ask us that question again as we will tell you when we think that it is time for you to know."

At his request I even promised Dr. Kubilius that I will not ask Dr. Carmichael any questions concerning my heart and now I already regret that I ever made this promise. I would like to ask about this spell I had at home and discuss my condition with these doctors as I am curious and do believe that it would be better for me to be told the truth.

Dr. Carmichael had me in his office this morning and he told me many things and I reluctantly kept my promise and refrained from asking any questions.

The doctors wanted to keep me in the hospital for about two weeks longer to do more tests but I explained to Dr. Carmichael that I had not told my family about this heart condition and if they kept me in longer than the two weeks my Mother would surely become suspicious so I was allowed to come home today. However, Dr. Carmichael warned me that I must rest with my feet elevated several times a day if I wish to live for another twenty years and then he gave me some pills that I have to take three times daily.

Summer 1954

I continue to see Dr. Carmichael regularly concerning my heart but otherwise am leading a rather normal sort of life although I have developed a severe case of hay fever so do a lot of wheezing and sneezing which can be very unpleasant at times.

Tuesday, October 26th, 1954

I was in Ottawa to have a checkup from Dr. Carmichael and then I went over to the Preventorium to see Miss Clement and friends. Miss Clement was pleased to see me and then she asked if I was in the mood to do a good deed. She said that Miss Evans is seriously ill in the Perley Home in Ottawa South and that she knows a visit from me would please her. Miss Evans had been our night nurse at the Preventorium for many years.

Miss Evans was in a bright mood when I arrived at the Perley Home and she was delighted to see me. We chatted about many things and she asked numerous questions. And then she wanted to know if I was wearing a dress. When I replied that I was wearing a skirt and a blouse her face lit up. Though Miss Evans is now nearly blind she explained that if I would go and stand in front of the window she would be able to see me quite clearly. She said that in all the years that I had spent in the Sanatorium she had only seen me in pyjamas and would love to see what I look like when I am dressed up. As I stood in front of the window Miss Evans asked me to turn this way and that way until I began to feel like a model at a fashion show.

We had a very pleasant visit and I am really pleased that Miss Clement asked me to go and visit Miss Evans.

Friday, April 1st, 1955

Dr. Beamish started me on hay fever injections today and Miss Brown will be giving me two shots a week for a while. I sure hope the serum will stop all this.

Wednesday, August 24th, 1955

Ralph and Milly dropped Anne and me off at the Ottawa Exhibition Grounds and we had a wonderful time. However Anne's day would have been ruined without a ride on the Ferris Wheel and since she did not want to go up alone I finally mustered up the courage and accompanied her on this ride. Then Anne's day was made when we were high up in the air and my day was made when my two feet were safely back on the ground. We ate well and it was really one great day of fun.

CHAPTER TWENTY-FOUR

DREAMS FULFILLED - LOVE, MARRIAGE AND A SON

September 17, 1955 – 1960
Twenty-Eight Years, Eleven Months – Thirty-Four Years

Saturday, September 17th, 1955

Harry Flannigan phoned to ask me if I would go with him to the Metcalfe Fair this afternoon and help him to celebrate his 34th birthday. I went and we had a nice time. My family has known Harry for several years and I was introduced to him while the men were exchanging fish stories back at the Rideau River one day when we were there on a picnic.

Monday, September 19th, 1955

Nick is home on a few days leave from the Air Force so the two of us walked down the road and we measured off several lots with a two hundred and ten foot frontage to each lot as Mother is going to give a lot to each one of her children. After Nick has all of the lots marked off and numbered, we will draw a number from inside a paper bag and the number drawn will be our lot.

Monday, September 25th, 1955

I received a letter from Father Campeau telling me about his trip to Rome. He enclosed a picture of the Pope which has his blessing and my name on it. This token gives me great joy.

Sunday, January 1st, 1956

Harry took me to see *Prince Valiant* at the Kemptville Theatre last evening and then he came home and visited with my family.

Anne is a curious twelve year old and her greatest concern and worry today is whether or not Harry kissed me last night to wish me a Happy New Year. We aren't telling.

Monday, January 9th, 1956

The circulation in my hands and feet has been acting up lately and sometimes a finger or a toe will go numb and turn completely white and waxy. When I was at the doctor's for my allergy shot this afternoon I told Dr. Beamish about the problems that I am having with my circulation and he started me on Priscoline and I am supposed to see him again in a few days.

Winter 1956 continues

Dr. Beamish monitored the amount of Priscoline that I am receiving for my 'Raynaud's Syndrome' so the proper dosage can be established for my condition.

Friday, July 6th, 1956

Harry took me to see the 'pig races' that were held in Kemptville this evening and it was a very comical performance as pigs sure don't understand what racing is all about. The races were part of the activities celebrating Kemptville's Centennial.

Saturday, October 20th, 1956

Harry and I were married by Father Quinn in Holy Cross Church in Kemptville at nine-thirty this morning. The wedding was a small one and consisted mostly of relatives – the Flannigans, Rainas, McGoverns and Ellards. Father Louis Campeau and Miss Irene Clement also attended and they added so much joy to the occasion.

Mother baked our wedding cake and the reception was held at home.

1956 Continues

After the wedding trip we settled down into a normal married life. My Disability Pension was discontinued as it was now felt that Harry would be able to support me.

Then in 1959 we adopted an extremely active two and a half year old boy and things were quite different from that day on.

The day that we were introduced to Billy we first made a visit to church and asked God to help us in the raising of this child and to assist us to be good parents.

Billy was a dear little boy and so full of love and frustrations. We were awakened many times during the nights when Billy would have nightmares and wake up sobbing, "I want to stay here, don't let them take me away."

Thus we spent many hours at his bedside assuring him that he was ours to keep and never again would have to be moved.

Six months later the day finally arrived when Dr. Spence prepared the adoption form and Billy asked him what the papers were for. When given a wonderful explanation from Dr. Spence, Billy became very excited. And after that Billy would proudly tell our visitors, "I can't go away with you because I have papers that say I belong here forever."

We soon became a close knit family and did many things together so it was a great blow when Harry took a sudden heart attack in 1960 and was in the hospital for six weeks. This illness proved to be very upsetting for Billy but we did manage to pull ourselves together again. However, we now had added worries as Harry and I both had serious health problems.

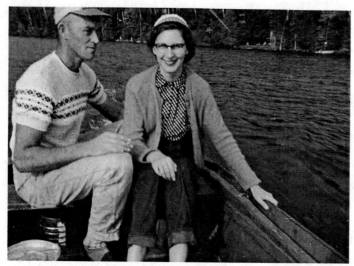

Summer 1956. Harry Flannigan and Clara Raina on a fishing expedition.

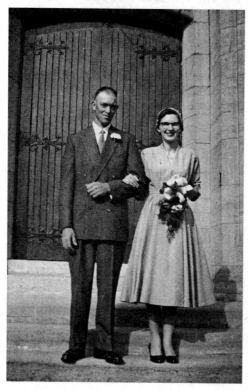

October 20, 1956.
Clara Raina and Harry
Flannigan Wedding
Day, Holy Cross Church,
Kemptville, Ontario.

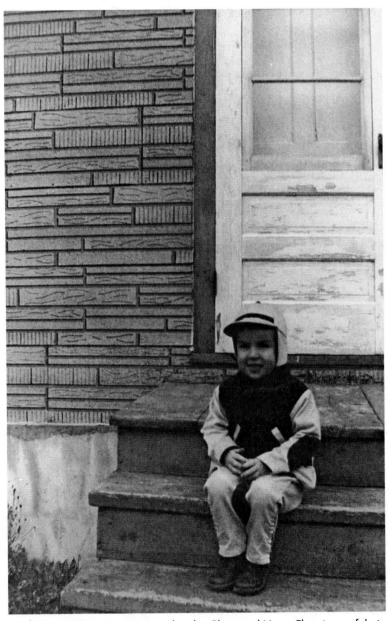

November 1959. First picture taken by Clara and Harry Flannigan of their wonderful new son, Billy Flannigan.

CHAPTER TWENTY-FIVE

DOCTOR CARMICHAEL DIES

Monday, January 9, 1961
Thirty-Four Years

While listening to the news on the radio this morning, I learned that our beloved Doctor Carmichael had died yesterday. This came as a great shock to me as I had not heard that he was ill.

When Ralph was at the San for a checkup last month he had met Dr. Carmichael in the hall and he had asked Ralph about me. Then Doctor Carmichael reminded Ralph a second time to be sure and give me his best regards. There seemed to be an urgency in his request so Ralph phoned me as soon as he arrived home to give me Dr. Carmichael's message.

Even though Dr. Carmichael had officially retired in 1955, I continued to have my medical examinations from him until the present time. Whenever I was due for a checkup I would just write a note to Dr. Carmichael. He would then show my letter to the other doctors and they would allow him the use of their office. Doctor Carmichael said that he needed the note from me so the other doctors would know that I still had faith in his ability and really wanted him to look after me.

I always enjoyed going to Dr. Carmichael after his retirement as he was no longer in a rush and he would relate many interesting stories. His memory was extremely keen and his mind never became dull. He would tell about his early years in the medical profession and about the day that he had decided to become a doctor. On that particular day he entered his home, removed his carpenter's apron and informed his mother that he would really like to become a doctor. His mother replied that if he wished to be a doctor, then by all means he should be one and that was how it all began.

Another time he told me about his class reunion. There were only three doctors left, including him and there was sadness in his voice as he spoke. He indicated that his turn could come at any time but as long as he was around that he would be pleased to give me my checkup if I thought that he was still capable. I assured him that I had complete faith in his abilities and appreciated having my checkup from him. I found that he was a brilliant man always, including the last times that I saw him.

Dr. Carmichael would often speak about his daughter Jean. He was so proud of her.

Memories continue to flash through my mind and I still feel numb with the sad news. I remember how Dr. Carmichael used to tap his one foot on the floor whenever he thought 'bad news' even though he might have been speaking of pleasant things at the time. I never did tell anyone when I discovered the meaning of his 'foot tapping' but after each tapping session I would begin to question him as I never had peace of mind until I knew what the bad news was and only then would I be able to come to terms with myself regarding the situation. On these occasions Dr. Carmichael would usually try to avoid a direct answer and brush me off by saying that I ask the darndest questions or that I was just too nosey.

However, there was the day when he did become very upset with one of my questions and as he sat there gazing directly at me he answered my question with another question, "Clara, I *want* to know, *why* did you ask me that question?" I just sat there dumbfounded as I was not about to say, "because I *know* there is something wrong when you begin tapping your foot on the floor."

After moments of silence Dr. Carmichael finally began to move everything from one side of his desk to the other side – one article at a time. And when he was all through I was still speechless so the doctor spoke once more. "Clara I don't know what made you ask that question – and besides there isn't any need for you to know at this time – but the answer to your question is – yes."

I was quite upset over this incident as Dr. Carmichael all of a sudden looked as though he had aged about ten years and I sensed his thoughts as surely as if he had spoken these words, "No doctor should ever allow himself to worry this much over any one patient as I have allowed myself to worry over Clara."

I really felt miserable as I walked out of Dr. Carmichael's office that day.

Then there was another time when Dr. Carmichael was in one of his jovial moods and one of the patients asked him a question pertaining to himself. He winked and grinned as he replied – "Why don't you ask Clara. I think that she could tell you more about me than I can tell you about myself."

And now a comical little story about our departed doctor. I was at home at the time and had gone back for a checkup. Just as Dr. Carmichael was about to call me into his office he spotted a wedding party coming down the hall heading toward the desk to obtain their pass to visit one of the patients. Much to Dr. Carmichael's disappointment he was expecting a very important phone call so could not leave his office at that time. Thus I was instructed to hastily head down the hall and to carefully check over the wedding party, and to see if the bride was beautiful and also find out who they were coming to see.

I immediately set out and carefully followed all instructions as directed. After the wedding party had left with their pass, I approached the desk and obtained the information from the girl on duty. We shared a few chuckles, and agreed that things were never dull when Dr. Carmichael was around.

Then I returned to Dr. Carmichael's office with all the information and continued chuckling to myself as I was struck with an almost uncontrollable urge to tell him that it must be the environment that makes me so nosey when I ask all those questions that he doesn't appreciate me asking him.

Dr. Carmichael had been the Superintendent at the Royal Ottawa Sanatorium from 1926 until his retirement in 1955.

The new building that had reached near completion when I was discharged in 1952 was later named the Carmichael Building in his honour.

Harry took me to Dr. Carmichael's wake in Ottawa and I really appreciated getting there as it was an extremely cold day. Dr. Carmichael looked so natural lying there in his casket that I almost expected him to sit up and speak to me. And as I sadly stood there viewing the body I realized that now one of 'The three Great Cs' was gone.

I still keep in touch with the other two 'Great Cs', Father Campeau and Miss Clement, and I hope that they will live in good health for many more years.

CHAPTER TWENTY-SIX

MORE ABOUT FATHER CAMPEAU

Many years have passed since that day in 1945 when Father Campeau and I made our agreement that I would become his little co-missionary. Father was newly ordained when he first came to us at the San in 1944. He was still so young but so wise. He seemed to be able to read our very souls, if one can use such an expression.

No matter how ill we were, Father Campeau never seemed to be appalled at our outward appearance but instead his eyes always showed love, compassion and forgiveness. Father possesses a keen sense of humour and he can say more with a few words and expressions than many priests say with a long sermon. With his many attributes, the Protestant and Catholic patients alike all loved Father Campeau.

Father has served as hospital chaplain for more than half of his years in the priesthood. The hospitals consisted of the Royal Ottawa Sanatorium, The Ottawa Civic Hospital and the Ottawa General Hospital. Then on the Quebec side there was the Sacred Heart Hospital in Hull.

Father also served as assistant priest at St. Bonaventure in Ottawa and at Chenéville, Quebec. There were also a few years put in as the Parish Priest at Papineauville, Quebec.

As the years fly by I have been very neglectful in regards to saying prayers for my special priest but in spite of my many failures and shortcomings I do believe that my life has been much richer than it would have been if I had never known Father Campeau and if we had never made our little agreement.

In these times when many people think so lightly of their religious duties I too may have fallen by the wayside. Then something deep down inside keeps reminding me that Father Campeau is still counting on my prayers and sacrifices. Going to Mass is important as I always offer a part of my attendance at Mass and Holy Communion for Father and his many undertakings.

Among the photographs displayed in our home are a couple of snapshots of Father and these pictures remind me to say a few short prayers for him as I go about my daily chores. There are a number of different prayers that I say but I think that my favourite one still is "God please love, bless and protect Father Campeau. Keep him free from sin and help him to succeed in all his undertakings and to bring many souls back to God."

I am sure that priests must need to have a great deal of patience, especially the ones who spend much of their time caring for the sick and listening to their problems.

As I think of Father Campeau and of his gruelling work I hope and pray that God is close by to comfort him when he experiences some of his own heartaches.

One of my favourite religious pictures is the one of Our Lord's Agony in the Garden. We all experience our own little agonies at various times and I think that this picture enables me to a small degree to appreciate what Our Lord has suffered. I would like to think that Father Campeau is not left alone in his times of stress but that God makes his presence felt close by.

There have been times when I was deeply troubled and how I longed to see Father at those times as I knew that just seeing him would put my mind at peace again. However, this was seldom possible and I would have to work things out on my own. Sometimes God seems so far away and totally unaware of my very existence.

I think that these are the golden opportunities that are given to us. We can either sit up and take notice and emerge as a better person or we can lay back and give in to self pity. I have experienced both – a few successes and many failures. There were many opportunities when I might have gained a few merits to help Father Campeau's work but instead I just sat back grumbling and feeling sorry for myself. At those times a good swift kick in the derriere may have helped to smarten me up a bit.

Father Campeau and I have had an occasional visit over the years and these visits have been some of the happiest moments of my life. We also keep in touch by correspondence which is a great comfort to me.

My deepest and fondest wishes for Father Campeau are for his happiness and a sense of accomplishment in his work caring for his beloved sick and all of his other responsibilities.

God please always watch over my special priest in a very special way!

CHAPTER TWENTY-SEVEN

HAPPY MEMORIES

Harry, Bill and I have many happy memories of the numerous things that we did together as a family throughout the years.

Our camping trips consist of some of our fondest memories. Camping at Bon Echo was one of our favourite spots and we often took Mother and our nephew Paul Raina, who is Ralph and Milly's son, along with us when we went there to camp. Occasionally both Mother and Paul would come along on the same trip which made for a crowded tent and cause for much laughter. Billy was a holy roller in his sleeping bag and we never knew where he was going to roll or whose territory he was going to invade in his sleep.

There is a difference of six months in Paul and Bill's age and Granny Raina often took it upon herself to entertain these two active boys. Feeding the chipmunks and squirrels was one of their favourite pastimes except that we always seemed to run out of peanuts – that is until Granny came up with a great idea on how to extend the animals' mealtimes. Mother took the hooks off a couple of fishing rods and then she tied a peanut at the end of each line. Now the boys were ready for action and this new venture provided us with an endless amount of laughter. The squirrels' first reactions were looks of bewilderment and frustration and then came enlightenment as they began to chew through the line and run off with the peanut. Some squirrels learned much more quickly than did others so it was always very interesting to note how each one would react to this little ploy.

On several occasions two or more related families would camp in the same park and we always had a good time sitting around a campfire at night and participating in daytime activities. There were hikes, swimming and fishing and the usual tales about the fish that got away.

As a child Billy always enjoyed picking wild flowers. When his bouquet was picked he would hold the flowers behind his back, then bow graciously and say "Mon Cheri" and present me with his token of love.

While out hiking in a remote area on one of our camping trips Billy spotted some wild flowers and in his excitement he became lost. We became frantic but did find him in a matter of minutes, tear-stained and clinging to his flowers. Needless to say, that was one of my most treasured bouquets.

Another sentimental memory concerns a fishing trip the three of us took to a stream in another remote area. Harry was bound and determined that he would catch at least one fish before we headed back to camp. However things were not looking too promising when all of a sudden his rod bent and there was a fish on the line. Harry was elated when the fish was landed on the shore, but alas, the fish got off the hook and was heading down the muddy embankment toward the water. Billy lunged forward in an attempt to grab the fish but as it was even quicker than Billy was they both ended up in the water. The water was quite deep but Harry was able to pull Billy out as soon as he surfaced. Billy was sobbing and trying to speak all at the same time saying "I tried to save the fish for Daddy because he wanted to catch one so badly." We were several miles from camp and since Billy was totally drenched we made a hasty departure without any fish but it was a memorable family experience.

Billy's act of valour continued to amaze us as he never would touch a fish or a worm until that day nor did he ever want any part in the sport of fishing.

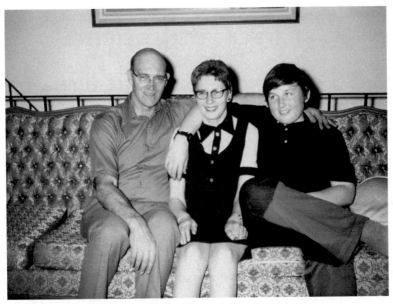

1972 – Harry, Clara and Billy Flannigan.

CHAPTER TWENTY-EIGHT

IN SICKNESS AND IN HEALTH

Doctor Dennis Jones has been our family doctor here in Kemptville since 1960 and I feel that his wise judgment and good care has been instrumental in prolonging my life and sustaining reasonably good health for what I consider well beyond my life expectancy.

Mrs. Marva Milne, the nurse at Dr. Jones' office, administers my allergy shots and she is always pleasant and very efficient. The patients always receive a warm greeting from Mrs. Isabel Taylor who works in the doctor's office.

Dr. Jones removed Billy's tonsils in the Kemptville and District Hospital when he was four years old and he was Billy's idol.

At about age nine Billy was in the Civic Hospital for throat surgery to remove a thyroglossal fistula. This operation was totally successful after Billy had gone through years of discomfort with this condition before having surgery.

In 1969 I was hospitalized for a few days in the Kemptville Hospital to receive treatment for a heart problem. Later Dr. Jones arranged that I be examined by a cardiologist in Ottawa. Dr. Evan Patrick was very easy to speak with and he took the time to explain his findings to me. Dr. Patrick said there was a scar on my heart muscle which he believed was caused by tuberculosis. I have been on heart medication since that time as well as being treated for the Raynaud's condition that involves my hands and my feet.

Things were going reasonably well in our household until the spring of 1971. Then so much seemed to go wrong.

I did have cystic mastitis in both breasts for quite some time but I had never mentioned this problem to the doctor as the lumps would always disappear after a short time. However, it suddenly occurred to me one day that there was a large lump, unlike the others, that had been there for a long time, possibly for several months. With this realization I lost no time in going to see Dr. Jones. He immediately began to make arrangements for a biopsy to be performed. Taking into account the condition of my heart and lungs the surgery would take place at the Civic Hospital in Ottawa.

Harry became very quiet when told about my checkup and I suspected that he was extremely upset. Two days later he took a serious heart attack while at work in Ottawa. He was rushed to emergency at the Civic Hospital and was admitted into Intensive Care.

My surgery was postponed until Harry was out of Intensive Care. Then shortly after, I was admitted into the Civic Hospital under the care of Dr. Norval Williamson.

I was examined by Dr. Evan Patrick, the cardiologist and then the two doctors consulted with each other to reach a decision.

Dr. Williamson explained to me that if the lump was malignant the breast would be removed when the biopsy was performed the next morning.

I didn't sleep too well that night as so many thoughts raced through my mind and I wondered!

"How could I have been so stupid not to have realized much sooner than I did about this one large lump that stubbornly remained in my breast? Now if I have cancer will the doctor be able to remove all of it? Will my heart and lungs be able to withstand the surgery?

If I do have cancer will Harry be able to accept me this way? What about our son? What will happen to him if I don't make it? He is only fourteen years old. I love them both so very much."

I worried most of all over Bill. At the time of his adoption we were cautioned that illness in the family could be very upsetting for Bill because of an incident in his early childhood when he had to be removed from a very happy foster home due to an illness in their family.

When I awoke in the recovery room after surgery and learned that I still had my left breast I was ecstatic. That meant there was no cancer. The surgeon and cardiologist both expressed their joy and I knew that I was very fortunate to be in the care of these fine doctors.

During our stay in hospital Harry and I both received excellent care and the nurses alternated taking us in wheelchairs to visit each other.

I was discharged one day before Harry came home. And as the results of these illnesses we were now a family with badly frayed nerves and I felt that outside help would be necessary to get our household running smoothly again. Thus arrangements were made for the three of us to receive 'Family Counselling' through the Children's Aid Society of Brockville, Ontario. We were most fortunate in obtaining this assistance from Mr. David Rice as the three of us liked this gentleman and were able to communicate freely with him. Mr. Rice was always very patient and serious when necessary but at the same time possessed a marvellous sense of humour.

The three of us each benefited in our own way from the many sessions of 'Family Therapy' that we participated in. Mr. Rice will always be remembered as a good friend who helped us in our time of great stress.

Harry made a good recovery from his heart attack and returned to work after a few weeks' sick leave.

I continue to be troubled with cystic mastitis and had to have two more biopsies. The right breast was done in 1972 and the left breast again in 1976. I have been very fortunate as there never has been any cancer. Dr. Norval Williamson did all three biopsies in the Civic Hospital and I always received the best of care. Each time Dr. Williamson would call Dr. Patrick in for consultations and I always had complete confidence in their decisions. They are both truly wonderful doctors and the very finest of human beings.

Twice yearly I return to Dr. Williamson's office and the patients are greeted in a pleasant manner from both him and Dorothy Black, his nurse.

On December 28th, 1978, Bill was married and, like most parents I suppose, we were a little saddened to see him leave home.

Then on October 31st, 1979, our dear Mother passed away very suddenly after suffering a massive heart attack. Every morning at nine I would phone Mother and we had our usual chat that morning. Mother said she had a rather uncomfortable night but felt better after getting up and planned to go to the bank with Ralph at 10 a.m. Before we ended our conversation Mother made a humorous comment so our last moments were spent chuckling at her remarks.

When Mother failed to put in an appearance at ten, Ralph hastened up to her apartment and he found Mother in great pain and very ill. An ambulance was called and Mother was rushed to Kemptville Hospital. Shortly after being admitted Mother went into cardiac arrest and passed away around noon.

Louis came from Red Deer, Alberta, to attend Mother's funeral. As we eight children stood around Mother's casket we shared our fondest memories of our beloved Mother.

In my autobiography I spoke mostly of my own illness as I did not know if my brothers and sisters wished to share their sickness with others who may eventually read my story. Now I will take the liberty to speak briefly of each one so you can more clearly understand how our dear Mother suffered for all her children. For each pain that we suffered I think that Mother's agony was even greater than our pains were.

Mother sat by and saw her husband and two sons die from tuberculosis. John, the oldest boy died in 1939, at age eighteen. Billy, the youngest boy, died in 1944 at age four. Mother was fifty-one years old when Dad died in 1952.

Mary, Ralph, George and Jim were in the Sanatorium with tuberculosis and as Mother admitted each child into hospital her tears were many.

Each one in turn had their dreams shattered when struck down with tuberculosis. Jim was always so sports-minded and we recalled how Mother had wept when at age fourteen Jim had to enter the Sanatorium shortly after the death of our father.

Louis and Dominic (Nick) escaped tuberculosis and both had spent years in the Air Force. Both were always kind and generous to the ones who were ill. When those who were ill recovered they too were very generous to the ones who were ill.

Anne, the tenth and youngest child never did contract tuberculosis and she was a comfort and joy to Mother as the two had shared several happy years together after all the other members of the family had left home.

Then there were the four years of mental suffering from 1932 to 1936 I mention in Chapter Two, 'Please Allow Me to Forget'. Mary covers those years in an excellent book that she has written, called 'We Have Written'. Mary, Nick and Anne have a real gift for writing. I can't help but envy them as I have been very frustrated many times while trying to write my autobiography as I knew what I wanted to say but couldn't find the right words to express my feelings and inner emotions.

Thus we all reminisced and wept over our dear Mother but in spite of our grief not one of us could wish Mother back as she had told us many times how she had fervently prayed that God would take her quickly when it was her time to go.

In spite of our great loss I feel that Mother is still very close to me and I am sure that it will always be this way.

Mother only received a grade three education as she was kept at home to help to care for her ailing mother. However, she was a wise little lady and I would like to share a copy of a personal will that she left to her family. This letter was read at Mother's funeral, as well as a poem that Anne had written for Mother on her last birthday, which follows the letter here.

March 15, 1969.

My Will to My God and Creator.

Who has been my Companion hope
and Comfort, when at times I felt
so lonely and forsaken, And I thought
I could go on no longer, Oh my God
you were near to Comfort me, Oh
I could feel your touch and new
hope and strength, to keep up my
strength for the sake of my husband
and children, I thank my God for all
you have given me, You have dried
my tears, You picked me up when I fell
down, You gave me light when all
seemed so dark, In sickness and in
death of my beloved once, you gave
me faith, and Courage, For all you have
given me, I give to you my sinfull
soul, If you will take it, with all my
love, to the ground my body,
And my dear children to guide and
inspire, Please dear God do not let
them stray away from you.

My Will to My God and Creator, written March 15, 1969, by our beloved
Mother, Elizabeth Hepp Raina.

Forgive them for their short comings,
Guide them and help them to be of
good faith, be their Comfort and
strength, To give good examples to their
mates and children,
To my dear children I leave all
my earthley goods, love and blessings
to love one another, overlooking faults
and shortcomings, above all be just in
your transactions, Don't weep for me
my beloved children, You have been
kind and considered, I injoyed you and
loved you so very dearly, Pray for me and
forgive me if I have failed, I have tried.
but we all make mistakes, So again I
beg you not to weep. But thank God
for all good things he has given me,
and also to you,
Thanks again my dears.
Forever mother and mother inlaw,
Granny,
God Bless and keep all my children
and Grand-children, Granny. Mother
xxxx/x xxxx x xxxxx xx xxxxx xx xxxx

MOTHER

How does it feel to be seventy-nine
To be celebrating a great passing of time?
How does it feel to have experienced so much
To have been a strong influence on those you have touched.

How does it feel to have your children all grown
Healthy and mature and doing well on their own?
Do you really understand how your grandchildren care
About how special you are and having you there.

Is it all that important if hills take a bit longer
When your sense of humour and wit keep growing stronger?
Does it bother you that your hair has turned grey
Or do you know that we find it becomes you that way?

When you look into a mirror does it clearly show
The twinkling eyes and soft face and love that we know?
Is it difficult to accept that your hard work is done
That the time for leisure and relaxing has finally come.

Do you sometimes wish you could join the younger pace
While they envy you the surpassing of their hectic rat race.
How many years did you work as hard as the best
Can you appreciate now that you've earned time to rest.

When your children were babies and you were pushed at and tugged
Did you ever foresee how much you would be loved?
What does it feel like to be seventy-nine
To us, you are the most beautiful mother of all time.

Love from Anne to a Special Mom on her birthday
September 9, 1979

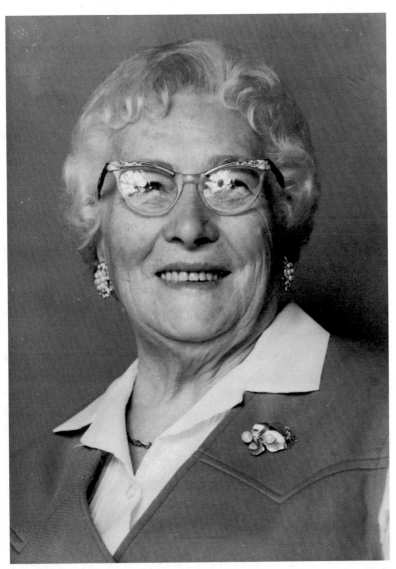

Our dear Mother, Elizabeth Hepp Raina.
Picture taken in 1977, at age 77 years.

The week prior to mother's death I learned that I had a fibroid tumour and thankfully I did not tell Mother about this health problem.

Then in late summer of 1980 my pap smear was positive and I was admitted into the Ottawa Civic Hospital. I had minor surgery on September 23rd and major surgery on September 30th, 1980. Dr. Irving Soloway removed a fibroid tumour (larger than a grapefruit) and did a complete hysterectomy. No cancer was found and I came through with flying colours. Dr. Soloway and both anaesthetists were great and did an excellent job.

My blood pressure was high and once again dear Doctor Patrick looked after my heart and my related problems. Doctor Patrick has two things going for him. He is a top rate doctor and does have a most delightful sense of humour. If 'Laughter is the best Medicine' holds true, then I was well medicated each time Dr. Patrick entered my room.

Once again I realized how many wonderful people there are in this world. The entire Medical Staff and care at the Civic was great.

Harry came often and was as kind as a husband could be. Also my son Bill and his wife Barb remembered me with attention and kindness. My sisters and brothers, in-laws, nieces and nephews were tops, all of them.

Father Louis Doherty was home on holidays from the States and he visited me in the hospital and said a Mass for my recovery. This was a comfort to me.

Last, but not least, dear Father Campeau once again was on hand on the day of major surgery. He also said a Mass for me and visited me a few times in hospital. Father Campeau was a tower of strength and comfort to both Harry and me during my stay in hospital.

God was indeed very generous to make all these things possible for me to be surrounded by all these wonderful people.

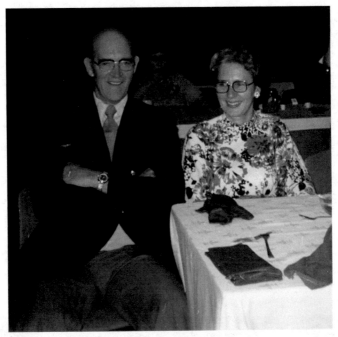

Harry and Clara Flannigan, October 15, 1977

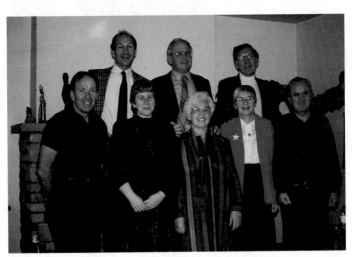

October 27, 1985.
Front Row: L to R. Nick, Anne, Mary, Clara and George Raina
Back Row: L to R. Jim, Louis and Ralph Raina.

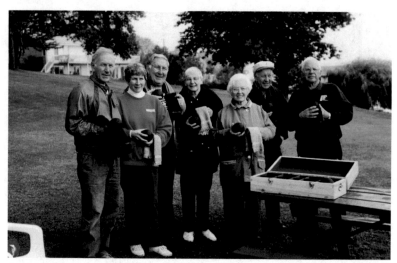

September 26, 1997. 'Raina Clan Getaway'
Left to Right: Jim, Anne, Ralph, Clara, Mary, Nick, Louis.
Such a Happy Time!

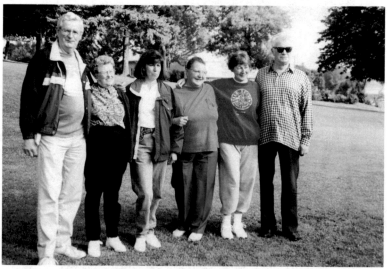

September 26, 1997. 'Raina Clan Getaway."
The Outlaws.

Left to Right: Grant Cameron (husband of Anne), Elsie (wife of Louis), Nancy (wife of Jim), Sonia (wife of Nick), Cathie (wife of Ralph), Ronald Rodgers (husband of Mary). It was a bright, squinting day!

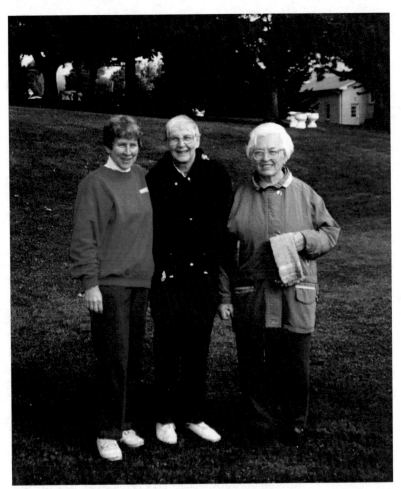

September 26, 1997. The Three Raina Sisters again.
Left to Right: Anne Raina, Clara Raina Flannigan, Mary Raina Rodgers

AFTERWARD

Clara's last notation for her book was about events occurring in September 1980. This Afterward is written in response to comments about Clara's book and questions about what happened in her life between 1980 and her death in May 1998.

Someone noted that Clara wrote in less detail of events following her years in the San. This was no accident on Clara's part. The story she wanted to focus on mainly was about the transition from child to woman within the confines of a medical institution.

Clara was forever grateful for all the extra years she had to live and never took them for granted or viewed them as anything but a great gift. Marriage and having a child were miracles she had dreamed of but had never thought of as being attainable.

Clara and Harry shared twenty-five happy years together. In September 1981 Harry had heart surgery, from which he did not, unfortunately, recover well. The following month our much-loved sister-in-law Milly died and this was a great loss for all of us. Milly's death was cause for much sorrow for our brother Ralph and their son Paul.

Harry's health continued a rapid decline and on December 1, 1981, Clara and Harry moved into an apartment in Ottawa to be closer to their medical team. Leaving their beloved country home at Kemptville was a great wrench but they could no longer look after their extensive property.

When I went to help them unpack the day they moved in, I found Harry to be seriously ill and feeling deep sadness that he could not help Clara with the work of moving and unpacking. A call to my brother Jim resulted in him taking Harry to emergency the next morning. Having spent one night in their new home, Harry never returned from the hospital.

On January 15, 1982, Harry faced his second round of heart surgery. He and Clara asked me to be with them before he went down for surgery. In our hearts we knew that he would not come through the surgery. Clara let Harry choose the path of saying last goodbyes and, following his lead, the two of them directed all their comments to each other through me. For example, Harry would say "Anne, I wouldn't want Clara to know this, but she has been the very best wife that anyone could possibly have and she has made me so very happy." Clara, in turn, would say "Anne, I would never have imagined that I could have had so many wonderful years with such a dear and loving husband but if he knew that he might become conceited." This gave me an opportunity to also tell Clara all the things I knew our family, nieces and nephews and I would want Harry to know about how much he was loved by all of us. This whole exchange took place with tenderness, smiles, hand holding, much laughter and a tangible feeling of intense love. Harry excitedly told us about the wonderful visit he had had with Bill the previous evening. The three of us also shared some quiet prayer time. Their hugs as Harry was wheeled into surgery were to be their last. A few hours later, Harry's surgeon came to the waiting room to tell us that Harry had not survived the surgery.

Clara felt the loss of Harry keenly but, just as she had adapted to the many other losses in her life, she remained a positive and happy individual. Her strong faith always brought her significant comfort.

Three months after Harry's death, their son Bill and his wife Barbara had their first child, Danny. Sixteen months later, Danny's little sister, Shannon was born. Clara was thrilled with the arrival of her two grandchildren. In time Bill and Barbara divorced, but Danny and Shannon continued to fill her life to overflowing.

In September 1986 our family suffered another loss in the death of our dear brother George. For so many years there had been eight remaining siblings and George's absence left a void for all of us.

Jim and his wife Nancy took Clara along with their family on numerous trips to Florida, each such excursion much anticipated by her. The year they arrived in Florida only to discover that Jim had forgotten to pack her luggage was a source of great amusement to all of them.

For a number of years quite a few of we Raina siblings and in-laws would go on an annual blueberry picking trip to Kirkland Lake. We're all berry picking fanatics and these were extraordinarily fun times for all of us. We picked berries in the wild from early morning to late afternoon, choosing to ignore signs of bears and shrugging off the occasional bear sighting. We cleaned the berries in the evening and then played bridge almost until it was time to get up at sunrise and head for the berry patch again. These jaunts were filled with laughter, jokes and teasing and were activities in which, at one time, Clara could not have participated.

In the summer of 1995, Mary and I took Clara on a train trip out west. We three sisters spent a month together, and included in that time was a lengthy visit with our brother Louis and his wife Elsie at their home in Red Deer, Alberta. We had great chats and explorations with their children and many of our western cousins. For Clara, this was a trip she had dreamed about all her life. It was the first time she had returned to the province of her birth and where she had spent, in her own words, "six of the happiest years of my life." Louis drove us to the homestead near Hanna, Alberta, now devoid of any buildings, where John, Mary, Ralph, Clara, Louis and George had started life. What a tug on our heartstrings to see the long row of offspring of trees that our father had planted when he started farming there when he came to Canada in the early 1900s. Standing there stately, with proud bearing, those trees seemed to signify the value of strong family roots.

Our day's adventure included a visit to the Wiese School, now abandoned, but echoing with the laughter of the young Raina children and their childhood friends. The whole trip west was a memorable experience.

Clara's son Bill and his wife Joan Chernes enjoy a wonderful life together. After they had been together for quite some time, it came to light in one of their visits with Clara that Doctor Pritchard, whom Clara had thought so highly of in the San, was actually a first cousin of Joan's mother. Clara was excited to hear of a relationship between one of her favourite doctors and her special daughter-in-law.

For the most part Clara remained reasonably healthy, notwithstanding the repercussions of her tuberculosis. She always had reduced breathing capacity, heart issues, circulation problems and, in later years, severe asthma. She spent her last years enjoying life. Nieces and nephews loved spending time with Aunt Clara. She developed an active social circle in her apartment building, enjoyed playing bridge and most of all she liked to talk, talk and talk.

Family gatherings at Nick and Sonia's, Ralph and Cathie's or any of our other homes were always outings to which Clara looked forward, and she also entertained us on many occasions.

Clara mentioned in Chapter Twenty-eight that Bill hated fishing and anything to do with fish. People do change! As an adult, Bill has become a dedicated and enthusiastic fisherman like his Dad had been. He has the pictures to prove that most of his fishing stories are true. We were laughing too hard to show Bill any sympathy at a family gathering at our cottage, when he stepped off a rock into what he thought was shallow water, only to be immersed up to his neck, in pursuit of a fish on his line. Clara would have chuckled to see a repeat of Bill jumping into the water when he was small to rescue a fish of his Dad's. And, being a good Mom, she would have been more sensitive to his plight than we were!

In September, 1997, the seven remaining Raina siblings and our spouses spent three days together at a resort on the St. Lawrence River, near Prescott, Ontario. Mary and Ron, Ralph and Cathie, Clara, Louis and Elsie, Nick and Sonia, Jim and Nancy, Grant and I shared treasured moments, complete nonsense, silly skits and made many new memories. The same old jokes got told, the in-laws were reminded how lucky they were to be part of our family and all of us reveled in appreciation for one another.

Ralph brought along a set of bocci balls our father brought with him from Italy. We held bocci tournaments between the Raina siblings and 'the outlaws' and there was lots of reminiscing about our parents and our three absent brothers. One evening Clara initiated a discussion with Mary and me about which one of our family members would be the next one 'to go'.

A couple of months later Clara started to feel unwell. In March 1998 she consulted a doctor and was diagnosed with stomach cancer. Although the doctors felt surgery was a major risk for her, with a possible outcome that she would spend the rest of her life on a respirator, she opted to take the risk and came through surgery with flying colours. She, along with the rest of us, was absolutely elated with the results. Just as when she had tuberculosis and highs were often followed by lows, such was the case now. While she was still in hospital it was discovered that the cancer had spread to her liver.

During Clara's brief return to her apartment after leaving hospital, one evening she asked my daughter Kelly Anne and me to help her choose her burial clothes. Kelly Anne and I will always remember the laughter that accompanied Clara's comments as we held up her various potential outfits from her closet, as she lay in her bed considering the options presented to her.

My husband and I had purchased a cottage near Perth, Ontario, in March 1998. We had bought it with a view to having family members visit often and we knew that Clara would thoroughly enjoy such a setting. We held our first family gathering there for the Raina siblings on Sunday, May 17. Although Clara was terminally ill, she agreed to come for the day. We placed a bed on the deck for her and, as always, we all had a wonderful time together. Clara kept repeating over and over, "This is a piece of heaven right here on earth. I am so glad to have seen it." Grant and I have often remarked how happy we are that Clara got to see the cottage at least once. While we had always envisioned her spending a lot of time there, we sense her presence often. It was there that I wrote Clara's eulogy.

Clara died in the Elizabeth Bruyère Centre on the evening of May 28, 1998. All of her siblings, many of her in-laws and nieces were with her to see her off. And, most importantly, Bill said a lovely goodbye to her. While a family member had been with her around the clock during the days preceding her death, we were all with her for the final few hours. At that stage she could no longer speak but could hear. We talked her through those last hours, and although her breathing was laboured, she smiled her awareness of our presence.

I consider it divine intervention that during this time it suddenly occurred to me that the best send-off she could possibly have would be for Father Campeau to give her the Last Rites. Surely it was God's will that I was able to reach Father Campeau and he was able to come to the hospital on such short notice. We had not told Clara he had been called and when he walked into the room her face just lit up. Although she could not speak to him, the connection between the two of them was palpable. They had shared so much over the years. It was with a heavy heart and obvious sadness that Father Campeau bestowed the Last Rites on his good friend and long-time co-missionary.

Soft music played, we were all holding or touching Clara, as we said our goodbyes and we spoke to her of all the people she had loved so much who were reaching out their hands to welcome her home. As she slipped away from our touch we rejoiced in the knowledge that she was being embraced by so many people who loved her as greatly as we did.

Clara's funeral was held June 1, 1998. Following this page is a tribute our brother Jim wrote and which he presented at her funeral. Following that is the eulogy which I wrote and gave at Clara's funeral.

Although Clara was seventeen years older than me, we were great friends. Along with many other common traits, we shared a fear of thunderstorms and a love of clipping newspaper articles. After her death when I was carrying out my task of sorting through all her personal papers and filing cabinets, it made me laugh to find, amongst her myriad newspaper clippings, numerous items that I had also clipped out of the papers.

But Clara, a newspaper headline that was missing because it had never been published was *Human Rib Found in Local Landfill. Police Searching For Rest of the Body.*

I had followed my sister's directions and done what I was told. Tucked safely into her casket was a little package. It contained 'Clara's Rib'.

CLARA

Prior to my sister Anne presenting the Eulogy, I wish to express what Clara has signified to me and how she inspired my life.

I remember on one of our trips to Florida I had Clara portrayed by a Caricature artist. Prior to the drawing the artist asked about Clara's personality, lifestyle etc. In an instant I replied that Clara was a **"MARATHON LADY."** "Draw her picture running," I said. Clara found this exceptionally humorous and we shared a great laugh.

Although my portrayal selection was humorous, there was a deeper significance. A winning "Marathon Runner" must possess determination and will power that far exceeds normal boundaries. Clara **"MY MARATHON LADY"** had these attributes in full measure and pursued her goals relentlessly. She carried on running long after experts expected her to waver and fall.

Clara's goals and race was not singular. Clara's marathon was a marathon of hope, generosity and unquestioned love and this belief conquered all.

In running through constant winds and rain the **"MARATHON LADY"** continually generated and exuded humour, love and happiness.

On Thursday evening at 8:30 p.m. the **"MARATHON LADY"** with her family cheering her on crossed the finish line and won HER gold medal.

James Raina

Eulogy for Clara Raina Flannigan

Monday, June 1, 1998

Some time ago my sister Clara asked me if I would speak at her funeral. I would like to preface my comments with a little anecdote I think will tell you a lot about Clara, and about our family in general.

A week ago Sunday evening when my husband Grant, my daughter Kelly Anne and I were having an extended visit with Clara, at one point Clara and I were visiting on our own and I asked her if she would like to hear what I had prepared to say at her funeral. Her response was an emphatic and enthusiastic "YES" and she was so happy and moved by what she was hearing. She was so touched that she had been given an opportunity that few people ever have to hear what will be said about them, and she said she would not change one word, but she hoped it did not make her sound too nice. It was an incredibly intimate moment of sharing for us.

When Grant and Kelly Anne came back into the room she was beaming as she told them she just loved what I had prepared. "But," she said to Kelly Anne, "my only worry is that I think your mom makes me sound too nice."

"Well Aunt Clara," Kelly Anne said, "you don't think this is what mom is really going to say. This is just the fake copy. What she's really going to say is at home. You really didn't believe she would be saying these sorts of things about you." Well Clara laughed and laughed and said, "Well, of course, I should have known better." The four of us had such a good laugh together.

But Clara, as you really knew at the time, what I read to you was the real thing and now all of us will share in thoughts of you.

Today we gather together to celebrate the life of Clara Flannigan.

If I would be asked to describe the credo by which Clara lived her life, the words of one of her favourite prayers, the Serenity Prayer, immediately come to mind.

"God, Grant me the Serenity to accept the things I cannot change; Courage to change the things that should be changed and Wisdom to know the difference."

As most of you here know, Clara's life was filled with many health related challenges, starting with her getting tuberculosis just as she was entering her teen years. This intrusion into her life led to her spending most of her teen years and into her twenties either in hospital or at home on the cure, with ramifications that would last her whole life.

During her adolescence she was well aware that the doctors never expected her to reach, let alone live, past the age of twenty-one. She knew there was no expectation that she would ever be able to marry or to have children.

However, her fighting spirit and her unwavering faith, nurtured by the tremendous love of her parents and nine siblings gave her the **courage to challenge and change these dire predictions.**

Last October Clara turned seventy-one years old. Each day of her life was filled with gratitude for this extra time she fought so hard for. Fifty extra years that she had never expected to have were truly seen by her as a miracle beyond her wildest imagination.

What does one do with fifty years one does not expect to have?

Well, Clara spent most of her time being generous of heart and generous of spirit and seeing the good side of others. She lived her life with dignity and humour. She loved to talk and loved to listen and enjoyed communicating with others, of any age, whether a young child or an elderly person. Friends and family were very important to her. Giving of herself was second nature to her. It was a quality that we all admired and one that could also make us chuckle.

Any time we visited her, Clara was constantly offering tea, coffee, "would you like a piece of cake, have some ice cream, let me open this bag of chips or candy." There were always some sorts of little trinkets for the nieces and nephews.

A couple of years ago she became adept at mixing together all sorts of conglomerations of cereals, nuts, candies – you name it, she had it. She got to know who liked what combination and at family gatherings, for goodness sakes, we almost needed a tractor trailer to haul in her BIG plastic containers of 'mix'. In fact, we were seriously considering getting her a cement mixer to help her in her endeavours.

It was the little pleasures in life that gave Clara her biggest joys and, although life dealt her a different hand than she would ever have chosen, she certainly always had the **serenity to accept the things she could not change**. And with that acceptance came her great boundless appreciation for her unexpected miracles.

She shared twenty-five years of wonderful married life with her husband Harry, until his death in 1982. And unquestionably the greatest joy Clara and Harry ever experienced was the addition to their household of their son Bill.

To Clara, the arrival of Bill was the ultimate unexpected gift she had hardly dared to dream could come true. Clara, Harry and Bill shared so many happy times together and if Houdini had ever spent time watching them he could have learned much more about magic.

You see, no one could match the ingenuity of these three when they packed up for their frequent camping trips – sometimes for two or three weeks at a time – loading their tent, camping gear, fishing equipment, food supplies for a few weeks (and you already heard how generous Clara was in that department) and still managed to save room to take Mom and often my nephew Paul along with them. If you have any doubt about the skills involved in this packing routine, you have to realize that the car they owned for an extended period of time was a little Volkswagon.

Clara's love for her son Bill has extended warmly to Joan and her daughter Kelsey and she happily welcomed them into her life.

Clara has also been a very proud grandma to Bill's children, Dan and Shannon. To you, Dan and Shannon, I would like to say that your grandma has so much love and so many aspirations for both of you. She believes you both can and will accomplish great things.

You may think I am making a mistake by saying that she "has" instead of "had" these feelings for you but there is no mistake. Even though your grandma has died, you will feel her presence in your lives in countless ways. She will be ever present for you and to you and her love will be with you always. She was and is so proud of both of you.

The last line of the Serenity Prayer is **"the wisdom to know the difference."**

When Clara became seriously ill recently, she again put up a tremendous fight. Again she had been dealt a hand definitely not of her choosing, but this time, **in her wisdom**, she knew there was a **difference** and came to accept that it was time to follow a new path – a path she has faced with *dignity, courage, hope, faith and with humour.*

It has been a privilege for all of us who know and love her to have shared with her in some small way her journey along this new path. We have cried, we have learned much and best of all we have laughed a great deal.

We were, of course, spending a lot of time with Clara. The day before Clara was to be admitted to Elizabeth Bruyère Palliative Care Unit, I was sitting and holding her hand and told her Jim and Mary would be spending the night with her. She laughed and said "Why don't a couple more of you stay and play bridge all night?" We've often done that as a family. It took only a few phone calls to bring five of we siblings together to spend the evening and well into the night at Clara's playing bridge. With a phone call from our brother Lou assuring Clara that he and my sister-in-law Elsie were leaving Red Deer the next morning by car to come and see her, we brothers and sisters and much-loved in-laws of Clara were all accounted for.

Although Clara was too ill to leave her bedroom she was smiling ear to ear and then the instructions to me started. "Anne, take the pecan pie out of the freezer and make sure Grant has some. There are macaroons in the freezer too, Nick loves those, and there are lots of soft drinks in the closet – are you sure you can find enough for everyone to eat?"

"Oh, and don't forget there are lots of containers of mix in the cupboard." What a lot of laughs and chuckles we all had together that evening.

Not long ago I saw in the newspaper a few short lines, author unknown, that I believe speak to us of our celebration today. They read like this:

To Those I Love and Those Who Love Me

Now that I'm gone, release me, let me go –
I have so many things to see and do.
You must not tie yourself to me with tears,
Be happy that we had so many years.

Clara, we have released you, not without difficulty, but with a great deal of love.

We believe absolutely that there are many things for you to see and do.

We also believe that Harry, Mom and Dad and so many of our family members have welcomed you with open arms. One of the last things your son Bill said to you, while giving you a big hug, as we saw you off on your journey, was that there was a family gathering waiting for you that was way beyond any of the family gatherings you enjoyed so much here.

We can't promise you we won't shed some tears, but we are indeed so grateful we had so many years.

Clara – fly free – and thank you for your love that will be with us forever.

Anne Raina

POSTSCRIPT

I have been asked by people who have reviewed the book to relate a little history of how those in the family who did not have TB were affected. These requests gave me pause for thought, as it is a question that Clara sometimes asked me.

Clara was always interested in other people's perceptions of things and she would ask me what it was like to be the youngest in this large family of people afflicted with tuberculosis. She wondered how I made sense of all that was going on in the family when I was small. While Lou, Nick and I were always very grateful to have never had to contend with TB, Clara knew that, even though we three never had the disease, the ramifications of TB in our family certainly would have impacted us. And, of course, logically it did. I cannot speak for Louis and Nick, but I do have many memories from when I was little of the effects of TB on our family.

When I was a child, if someone had asked me what tuberculosis was, I would have had to stop and really think about my answer because it was simply the way life was. However, if pressed, I would likely have responded that it was a disease that took most of my brothers and sisters and my father to a big hospital and that I could hardly ever get to see them. I would have said that tuberculosis meant that I had never met two of my brothers and I missed them terribly without having ever known them and that I often wondered what they were like. I distinctly remember as a child feeling a deep sadness when family members talked of John and Billy and I certainly experienced a feeling of loss where they were concerned.

Because nobody under 16 years of age was allowed in to visit, I would have said that when I went along with my parents to visit those in the San, I would stand alone on the lawn under the huge trees and try to find the window from which the voice calling "Ansie" was coming. Then I would peer up at whichever brother or sister was waving from the window and we would exchange some conversation. I was extremely shy when roommates of Clara, Ralph, George and then Dad looked at me through the windows of those big buildings. On one occasion Clara got permission to have me take a quick peek at her room when I was five, but I was too shy to go all the way up the big stairs with so many of her friends standing at the top beckoning me upwards. I am still sorry I did not ever see the whole inside of the building that was her home for so many years.

One time when I went to visit though, I was taken into one of those big buildings for an appointment. Dr. Carmichael administered the BCG (Bacillus Calmette-Guérin) to me, in the form of scratches down my back when I was four years old. My back was then covered with adhesive tape until the following week when, during a follow-up visit, the tape was removed. BCG was actually the TB bacillus, given to help a person build up antibodies to fight off TB. The results are that a person always has a positive skin test but, hopefully, does not develop tuberculosis. I always referred to Dr. Carmichael after that as Scratch Cat.

I could have said that when I was six years old I overheard the Public Health Nurse telling my parents that my Father had tuberculosis and that he would have to go to the San. I wanted to protest that they couldn't take him away too. I knew that now I would only get to see him through a window high up in a building. There would be no more long walks with me holding tightly to his hand. He walked so fast and I had to quickly skip along to match his steps. There would be no more thrill of him letting me hold the reins before he unhitched the horses and, with his guidance, walk the horses around a bit to cool them down. There would be no more trips to the sugar bush with him in maple syrup time or following him out to the fields when he was cutting hay and there would be no more times he would bounce me on his knee.

I might have told about the time when I was five and I took my doll along with me on the school bus. When I got on the bus, the usually kind school bus driver, whom we all liked, asked me loudly, "Does your doll have TB like everyone else in your family does?" My teenage brothers were upset when everyone on the bus laughed and I felt extremely uncomfortable with everyone looking at me and laughing. It was the defining moment for me when I suddenly realized there must be something unusual about TB to cause people to react in this manner. Until then, TB was just the way things were in my family. Being young did not prevent me from learning there was a stigma attached to tuberculosis.

I would have been able to say that I had already noticed there was a difference in how some people treated the family. When family members were home on the cure, there were periodic visits from the Public Health Nurse. I remember Ralph, very annoyed, and yet snickering as he held a book in front of his face when one of those nurses would pay a visit. And Clara tried not to laugh at Ralph's laughter. Although my mother was a meticulous housekeeper, this particular nurse would spread newspapers all over the floor in front of her as she entered our home, I guess to keep from getting TB germs on the bottom of her shoes.

And Clara had told us that when she first went to the San that she felt badly because some of her best friends stopped writing to her. Some of them later told her that their parents were afraid that there would be TB germs on the letters if Clara returned their correspondence.

Perhaps I would have explained that TB was the reason my parents looked so worried if we ever got a long distance phone call. There was a look of dread on my Mother's face anytime the operator told her there was a long distance call. When I was small, people did not make long distance phone calls without a very good reason. Such a call usually carried inevitable worrying news of some new health set back with one of her children.

I'm not sure if I would have told anyone that I spent a lot of time looking into the bureau and washstand which contained my big sister Clara's possessions in her bedroom that she used when she was home on 'the cure'. I always thought maybe I was doing something naughty, as I would carefully pull out the drawers, one by one, and just look at what was there. Sometimes Clara would ask Mother to bring her some particular article when Mom was going in to visit. Clara would tell Mom to ask me where the article was. She would tell Mom that even though I knew where every single thing of hers was, that nothing was ever disturbed or tampered with. As an adult, I think now that my frequent explorations of her things were about much more than simply being nosey. I believe it was a way for me to feel connected to a big sister whom I rarely got to see up close for months at a time.

I could certainly have described my excitement when a big brother or sister was at home on 'the cure'. Everyone followed precisely any directions that had been given by the doctors at the San to a patient coming home. When Clara was home we would gather in her room to visit and play games. Many a game of Sorry my brothers and I played with her, board set up on her bed. On her nightstand was a box that contained all her prayers that she said daily and during that time we did not intrude on her. If she was home in the winter she followed the fresh air routine of the San and I would run into her cold room early each morning to close her window before she got out of bed. I had a pair of blue pyjamas with little pink pigs on them that Mom had made me and Clara often said that my braids would be flying out behind me as I made the quick trek into her room. On her dresser was a pink container made of Depression glass, the lid in the shape of a dog, that held her bobby pins. Also there was a green dog, cracked and repaired, that held pins, buttons and sundry other small items. Both of those are now on the bureau in our spare bedroom.

What I could not have explained, because I did not fully understand this until I was an adult, was that the reason when I was little and throughout my childhood years that I absolutely did not want anyone to know when I was ill or in pain was because I knew that in my family if you got sick you went away to a hospital for a very long time. And sometimes you died. So at a very young age, without understanding the why, I became efficient at masking pain so others could not detect it. And I would become extremely angry if anyone suggested there was anything wrong with me physically.

Any time any of those in the San came home for a visit of a day or two was cause for great celebration in our family. All of us were so excited to be together and Mom always prepared a feast. Our parents, brothers and sisters simply loved sharing time together. Except for one summer day that is, when I was about four years old. Ralph and Clara were home for the day. While Mom was getting ready to serve lunch I was outside with my big sister and brother. Suddenly they 'spotted' chicken pox breaking out on me. They called Mom to come and look at the chicken pox. I was furious with them. Usually quite placid, I screamed and cried and kept yelling "I DO NOT have chicken pox, I DO NOT have chicken pox, THERE IS NOTHING WRONG WITH ME." Nobody could understand why having chicken pox upset me so much. I did not even know what chicken pox was and I did not understand then why it bothered me so much either, but I think I understand it now.

While I might have had feelings of guilt at telling this next episode, as a child I would have felt justified in my actions. Not so long after the chicken pox episode, I had a cold and Mom was going to give me cough medicine. It was not the taste of the cough medicine I was concerned about, but rather that it signified that I must have something wrong with me, to need the cough medicine in the first place. I vehemently denied needing it. While Mom turned around to get the bottle and a spoon, I quickly and quietly disappeared. Seeking an escape, I hid behind the chesterfield in our 'front room'. Mom called and called me and then I could hear my Father, my Mother and my brother Jimmy searching high and low for me. First upstairs, then outdoors all over, worriedly checking in the well, all through the barn and the surrounding area. Their voices sounded more and more frantic as time passed and I was nowhere to be seen and I could hear them deciding where next to search. I felt guilty for causing them worry but there was no way I was taking any cough syrup that I did not need. Suddenly, Jimmy happened to come in the front door and he knelt down to look under the chesterfield. With relief and triumph, Jimmy yelled "I found her." At the same time he reached in to pull me out. His next yell was not of triumph but one of pain "She bit me and my arm is bleeding." It is funny how you can't process some things as a child but they become plain as an adult. I was neither vicious, nor nasty and certainly did not have a bent for cannibalism and I would never have wanted to hurt my beloved Jimmy. But neither did I need any stupid medicine. And I did feel betrayed by my brother.

I would not have been able to explain that sometimes my decisions had painful results. One day after school, when I was five, I walked along the top of a rail fence. I lost my balance and fell off hard on to the dry, packed earth, landing squarely on my left shoulder. The wind was knocked out of me and there was excruciating pain in my shoulder. I rarely cried from pain and did not do so then. After I gingerly got up and gained my equilibrium, I gritted my teeth and did not tell anyone what had happened. The pain did not subside for days. Until I was well into my late teens, every time I ran or the weather was very hot, the pain in that shoulder was searingly intense. Nobody ever knew of my experience.

What I definitely could have said was that by the time I was four or five, I had come to the self-imposed conclusion that no matter what bad thing ever happened to me in life, it was of little consequence compared to what was happening to all those in the family who had TB. I always took the attitude that I could handle anything and next to TB nothing really counted. As an adult I know that my parents would have been most dismayed at my perceptions in this regard.

I would have happily told of one of the most exciting highlights of my young life. Jimmy took me skating behind our home one December Sunday afternoon in 1951. When we came back in the house, a number of my friends were there. My family had organized a surprise birthday party for my eighth birthday. This was my first birthday party ever and I was excited beyond words. My Father, who was at home dying, was confined to the front room of the house during these festivities. But after dinner, while my friends and I played *Ring Around The Rosy* in the kitchen, my Father came and stood in the doorway watching us. He looked so tall and handsome and, as our eyes met, he just seemed so pleased to see me having such a good time. That was just four months before he died. It is interesting that two of my best friends today were at that party and they both mention to me sometimes that they remember that party and my Father standing in the doorway.

I could have told about the really special memorable April Fools' Day of 1952, three weeks before Dad died. Mom told him there was a fox out in our yard. When Dad went to look and saw nothing there, he said "There is no fox out there." Mom replied, with her mischievous smile, "April Fool." My Father laughed, gave her an affectionate little pat on her derriere and said to me "Your Mother is so foxy." I loved that exchange between them.

I'm not sure if I could have found the right words to properly explain my perceptions of the period leading into my Father's death at home. The family gathered on a number of occasions, when Dad was haemorrhaging from the lungs. This was quite scary to see, and we were never sure if he would live through each such episode. We were also all together of course when Dad was administered the Last Rites. As the youngest, I spent a lot of time just watching the reaction of other family members. My Mother was always a tower of strength. In that room where my Father lay dying, there was so much life. There was a lot of praying, a lot of crying, a lot of talking and, perhaps most importantly of all, a lot of laughing. The room was filled with love. And my Father had a most radiant and peaceful smile through most of this.

On the afternoon of the last day of school in June 1952, two months after my Father's death, Jimmy and George had gone to pick strawberries in a large garden patch far back on our farm. While they were gone an unexpected violent thunderstorm erupted. Within minutes the wind was whipping the trees, rain was blasting down, lightning flashed and thunder exploded everywhere. Baseball-sized hailstones pounded our home and cracked windows. The noise was deafening. For the very first time in my life I saw fear on my Mother's face. It was not us she was worried about but she lamented "Oh no, George and Jimmy are out in this terrible storm." She kept saying "I pray they are safe, I pray they are safe." More than anything I had ever wanted in my whole life, I wanted to be able to take the worry away from Mom. Helpless to do anything for her myself,

I suddenly found myself imploring loudly "Daddy, please help us, Daddy, please help us." It was at that moment, as though I had been struck by a lightning bolt, I realized that Daddy was really gone. As soon as the storm settled a little, Mom and I ran back to the field where my brothers were. They had taken refuge in our old barn and Mom's relief on seeing them was best expressed in her emotional heartfelt words to them "Thank God you are safe." Prior to that day, I had liked thunderstorms. Since that day I have always been frightened of thunderstorms and it is only during a thunderstorm that I experience a feeling of helplessness. Actually, I hate storms. Having my surroundings over the years receive six lightning strikes, including one that resulted in fire destroying the top story of our home in 1971 when my children were young has not helped to change my feelings towards storms.

I probably would not have told what a time of great loneliness it was when I was seven to nine years old. From spring 1951 when my brothers Lou and Nick joined the Air Force and left home, through my Father's death in April 1952 and Jimmy's departure for the San in March 1953, the house seemed so empty. Four of the most important people in my life disappeared from home in such a short time and I remember walking down the stairs in the mornings and finding it so strange to have the rooms not bustling with the activity of many family members. My brothers had always been so good to let me follow them on their long hikes through the bush, visits to 'the swamp' to get turtles, long forays to pick wild raspberries, strawberries and blackberries and I missed them a lot. Each one of them played a different important role in my life and I liked spending time with them.

Although he was fourteen years older than me, Louis and I were great pals. People frequently told us how much we looked alike and I always felt so proud to hear that. Louis was called

Louie by many people and my only problem with that was that I could not pronounce my 'Ls' when I was young. I wore my hair in braids and Louie would toss me in the air, and threaten me, laughingly, "Anne, I'm going to hang you from the ceiling by your braids." I, delighted with this familiar routine, would squeal in feigned terror, "No, Ouie, Ouie, Ouie, don't hang me up by my braids." It was 'Ouie' who had me repeat to anyone who came to visit, "The lazy little lamb likes lettuce" because he knew what would come out of my mouth was "The yazzy yitte yamb yikes yettuce." I missed our special camaraderie. Nicky, ten years older than me, read to me, built snowmen with me and used to champion my causes and stick up for me if I needed it. When he took me for walks he had an uncanny sense where a porcupine would be high up in a tree long before we could see the tree or the porcupine. He was invariably right and, sure enough, there would be Mr. Porcupine. Nicky, Jimmy and I would skate in the fields on moonlight nights, slide down our hill and together eat green apples with salt when they were the size of large marbles. When Nicky left, so did Jimmy's sports team mate. Almost six years younger than Jimmy, I now learned something new. Jimmy was a great sports enthusiast and he needed someone to play with. I learned that I was such a good hockey player that I could easily be drafted into the NHL. I could catch a baseball like Babe Ruth. I knew I really didn't have those sorts of skills, but Jimmy's enthusiastic flattery was all the encouragement I needed to play hockey with him and catch a ball fired with such speed that you could hear the resounding echo as I caught it and my hand would turn fire red. This feat would bring gasps from Mother and Clara. I thoroughly enjoyed such activities. It was also Jimmy who kindled in me a love of poetry. Life was much duller with those three brothers gone.

Dad was no longer in the front room where I could pop in and see him. He was a strong presence and his smile had been so comforting. And I had given up my imaginary playmate,

Mabble (as in babble, not Mabel as in table), many years ago of course. I spent a lot of time wishing that I had a brother or sister my age. It was so nice having Ralph at home though and I had been aware of how kind and gentle he was with my Father when Dad was so ill. It was wonderful when Clara came home from the San for good the end of 1952. A highlight of our week continued to be the sound of the Colonial Coach Bus stopping at our laneway Friday evenings when Mary came home from Ottawa for the weekends. Whoever was home would meet her as she stepped off the bus and would reluctantly see her on the bus again on Sunday afternoon. We were always happy that George came often and of course we were so excited when Lou and Nick would get home on leave. We were all best friends in our family. Even with so many in the family, if one person bought a chocolate bar it was always divided into equal pieces for anyone who was at home, before the owner would take one bite. Mom was always there for us, to give a hug, to talk and listen. She and I were very close.

When I got a little older, I certainly could have said that the winter I was twelve presented cause for alarm in my family. When I became really ill with red measles, I could not understand why everyone in the family was so upset about the state of my health. My temperature hovered around the 104 degree mark for a few days and I was quite unwell. Our family doctor made house calls to see me. This was an illness I couldn't hide because the sight of food made me throw up and when Ralph brought me a big piece of sponge toffee as a treat and set it on my bureau, I shyly had to ask to have it removed because the sight of it made me sick. I was afraid of hurting his feelings but I couldn't look at that sweet treat. Mom and my brothers and sisters warned me that I had to take good care of myself because I was the same age as a lot of my siblings were when they got tuberculosis. Red measles had been the pre-cursor to the onset of pleurisy and TB for them. At 12 years of age, these concerns did not make much of an impact on me and I thought they were all being worrywarts. I was annoyed at having to miss school as nothing could keep me away from class. I certainly incurred the wrath of my family when, on the first day I was allowed downstairs, I ran out to the road to get the mail from our rural mailbox, without first putting on a coat, hat or snow boots. However, as I read Clara's book, it is totally clear to me why my family would have worried about my health at that time.

But now back to the present. One of the most emotional experiences for me in preparing this book was holding in my hand the last letter John wrote Ralph and Clara before he died. It filled me with such deep sadness and such an aching feeling of loss. Mom often told me that my son Mark, from the time he was a little boy, reminded her so much of John in the sense of how thoughtful Mark always was of my feelings and how kind he was to me. Mom said John had always been like that with her from when he was little and treated her with that same extra care as Mark showed me. My daughter Kelly Anne had a most unusual, incredibly adorable smile as a baby. Everyone used to ask me where she got her smile from. Mom would say that Kelly Anne's smile was identical to John's smile when he was a baby. While my children and I were going through myriad family albums to choose pictures for this book, I happened across a picture I had never seen before and it took my breath away. There sat Mom, holding one-year old John on her knee. Off the picture jumped Kelly Anne's smile at the same age. Kelly Anne, too, was astounded to see this picture. There was no denying this striking resemblance to her Uncle John when they were little. Even though I had never known John in person, it turned out I knew a little of him through my children.

Mom used to tell me how Billy liked to talk to me when I was a newborn in my crib and how excited he was when she brought me home from the hospital. I have always been sorry that he died just five months after my birth. I have no trouble remembering my Mother's deep feelings of loss and sorrow at the deaths of her eldest and youngest sons, and her husband.

But my Mother was, quite simply, the most remarkable and wisest woman I have ever known. She had a resilience and attitude that was unbreakable. Although none of us in our family has any singing talent, as already testified to by Clara, every single morning that I lived at home I awoke in the morning to the sound of my Mother singing in the kitchen. The sound of her voice was beautiful, reassuring, and uplifting.

Each of us were also greatly influenced by my Mother's ability to see the positives in life and maintain a good sense of humour and ability to laugh, in spite of all the illness and challenges she, my Dad, and the family faced. Consequently, she passed on her gift of great inner strength and courage to face life to each of her children. Both of my parents were strong individuals, loved nature and the outdoors and one of the first lessons Mom taught us was that there is something good in every single day, whether the beautiful sunshine in morning, the first ripe strawberry in summer or the sound of the Whippoorwill at bedtime. With each obstacle I have met I have always believed that if Mom could cope with everything she had faced then there was nothing too insurmountable for me to contend with. That is the way we all think in my family. As Clara has shown time and again in her book, the family history of TB never took that away from any of us.

Germ warfare, by necessity, took on a whole new meaning in our household. In spite of her constant vigilence and close attention to her family's welfare, and her heavy burdens, my Mother was innately a really happy person who was a lot of fun to be around. She was extremely intelligent, witty, and deeply cherished as a Wife and Mother and absolutely adored by her grandchildren.

The amazing strength and resilience of all my family members naturally enveloped me in my formative years and those traits became ingrained in me. In this way I was truly blessed in being given an example which helped me deal with adversity as, not tuberculosis, but multiple autoimmune disorders have been a major factor in my own life. These include, but are not limited to, Interstitial Cystitis (IC), Irritable Bowel Syndrome (IBS), Osteoarthritis, Fibromyalgia and Histoplasmosis of the left eye, resulting in loss of functional vision in that eye. Ongoing severe chronic pain is exacerbated by my intolerance for pain medications. The support of my husband and children and the powerful legacy of my family are my mainstay for coping with these medical challenges.

I definitely would have said as a child, and I would also say as an adult, that I had an extremely happy childhood. We all spent hours playing games together, going for walks, talking, sometimes all at once, sharing an appreciation of reading and books, and being thoughtful of one another. Our friends were always welcome and were treated as one of the family and they came often. Our home was a very happy home and love, laughter, teasing and pure joy with one another were the fabrics of my years growing up.

I am so grateful I never had TB. I wish, with all my heart, that nobody else in my family had had it either.

Anne Raina

ACKNOWLEDGEMENTS

It is with sincere gratitude that I express my appreciation to my husband, Grant Cameron, for his enthusiastic support and encouragement in my journey to bring this project of publishing Clara's book to fruition.

The insight of my children, Kelly Anne and Mark McGahey, has been invaluable.

In addition, I wish to offer grateful thanks to ...

- My sister Mary Raina Rodgers, my brother Ralph and his wife Cathie, my brother Louis and his wife Elsie, my brother Nick and his wife Sonia and my brother Jim and his wife Nancy for their support and interest as I finally was able to embark on the quest to fulfill my promise to Clara.

- My nephew Bill Flannigan for his encouragement and his help in finding pictures that I wanted for this book. We had fun searching through his Mom's albums together. Most of the pictures in the book are from Clara's albums and the rest are from my family albums.

- To the Royal Ottawa Mental Health Centre for their permission to use pictures of the Perley, Whitney and Carmichael Buildings from the story of the Royal Ottawa Hospital.

- My dear friends Isabel Dingwall Wilson, Bernadette O'Neill and Betty Forth. The exciting and thoughtful dialogue that followed their first reading of Clara's manuscript was a positive catalyst in motivating me onward with this project. Isabel re-read the manuscript numerous times and she has been an enthusiastic and trusted sounding board.

- My many other friends for their encouragement, some of whom have been friends since grade one and who often visited my home and know my family well.

- A number of persons who responded with alacrity and interest to my requests for assistance in procuring specific information I was seeking on tuberculosis. Thank you to Elizabeth Czanyo and Owen Adams of the Canadian Medical Association; Sue Riley of the Royal Ottawa Mental Health Centre; Louise McRae and Jessica Evans, Public Health Agency of Canada and Lori Royea of Ottawa Public Health.

- Susan Jennings and the other members of my writing group, and the members of my book club, The Ramsgate Literary Society, for their thoughtful comments.

- Travis Murphy, for his sensitivity and creativity in bringing to life my vision for the cover of the book.

- My publicist, Randy Ray, for his wise counsel.

- Dr. Peter Jessamine, Medical Microbiologist & Infectious Diseases Consultant, Divisions of Microbiology and Infectious Diseases, The Ottawa Hospital, General Campus, for his keen interest, support and generosity of time in following the journey of *Clara's Rib* from its onset.

- Dr. Bill Jeanes, Former Medical Director, Canadian Tuberculosis Association, for his ongoing enthusiasm and interest. His sharing of memories of his own practice in tuberculosis has been deeply enriching.

Clara Raina Flannigan was a child who was happiest when she was playing outdoors, collecting gopher tails and crows' eggs or playing baseball. She dreamed of going to Immaculata High School in Ottawa. Her long range goal was to get a good job and save money to buy a riding horse. Instead, at twelve years of age, she entered the Sanatorium with tuberculosis. She did not go to high school, get a job or buy a horse. She became an inveterate diarist, graduated from the school of hard knocks with honours and banked her positive outlook in order to buy life.

Although losing much, Clara always felt she was a winner. She was happily married for twenty-five years and she and her husband Harry adopted a son, Bill, who was the light of their lives. Family was extremely important to her.

Clara never forgot the many friends she made in the San, and the medical team who contributed so selflessly to her wellbeing.

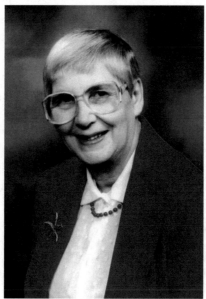

Clara Raina
Flannigan

Anne Raina worked for many years in the public and not-for-profit sectors. She was a senior executive with a national disability organization when struck with a disabling autoimmune disorder herself.

She has been writing poetry, skits and short stories for friends and family since she was a child and she has two children's books in the works. Although she has been published in magazines and newspapers, co-writing Clara's Rib is her first adventure in publishing a book. Anne is in high demand as a speaker, with a full schedule of speaking engagements. She was a keynote speaker at a large TB Conference in Toronto in November 2012 (TB: Making a Difference) and she has spoken at the Saranac Lake Laboratory Museum in New York State.

Her daughter, Kelly Anne McGahey, and her son, Mark McGahey, live in Ottawa. Her step-son, Stefan Cameron, lives in California.

Anne lives with her husband, Grant Cameron, in Ottawa.

Clara's Rib available at: www.anneraina.ca & www.clarasrib.ca

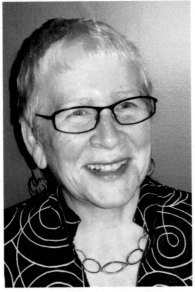

Anne Raina

About the Cover of
Clara's Rib

Enthusiastic comments and questions about the cover of Clara's Rib have prompted me to offer an explanation of how it came about. When I first considered co-writing and publishing Clara's Rib, definite ideas filtered through my mind for a cover design. To transfer my visual concepts to reality, I commissioned a highly talented artist, Travis Murphy, who was receptive to my suggestions. It was exciting to see what I had envisioned, bringing vibrancy and life to the cover, through his creativity.

Having a large maple tree on the cover held particular significance for me. There had been many huge trees on the expansive lawn at the Ottawa San. It was under those trees I would stand and wait for one of my many family members to call me through a window so we could talk a little. Because Clara spent months at a time in bed, often it was the trees that held her attention because that is all she could see. She speaks of the beauty of the leaves budding or changing colours.

So I wanted a tree, with the leaves reflecting the evolving of the four seasons and Clara's many years in the San. I asked Travis to depict a tree with a sturdy trunk, a tree that would not be blown down in a storm or break under a load of snow. This tree would endure and not suffer defeat, just as Clara had endured the storms of her life. For me, the branches of the tree also represent the ribs of a human being.

The opening picture in the book is a black and white photograph taken of Clara on her bed in the San, when she was 19 years old. Through the window behind her you can see the branches of one of the many trees. From the onset, I knew that this picture must be on the front of the book and I had sent it to Travis with that request.

Each time Travis sent me his latest version of the cover, it appeared on my computer screen in the open position, front and back covers in view. One morning at 4:30 a.m. I turned on my computer. There was Travis' latest work of art. I stood there, looking at the screen, while my eyes filled with tears. In my mind I had always seen the black and white photo on the front cover.

Travis, in his wisdom, had taken Clara out of that confining hospital bed, added sepia colour to the picture, and placed her outdoors, underneath one of our beloved trees, right where she should have been all along. Clara had been a child who reveled in being out of doors - that is where she had wanted to spend all her time. Although Travis did not know that, he intuitively sensed where she belonged.

I am grateful for the wonderful collaboration with Travis. Its always thrilling to me when people share their appreciation for the cover or ask about its origin.

Index

St. Francis Church (Ottawa, Ont.), 152, 171, 172
St. George's Roman Catholic Church (Hanna, Alta.), 1
St. Joseph's Church (Ottawa), 151
St. Joseph's Oratory (Montréal), 126
St. Margaret Mary, Sister, 103–4
St. Margaret Mary's Church, 200
St. Mildred, Sister
  anger at Clara for sliding down hill, 46–47
  belief in cod liver oil, 27, 46
  concern re Clara's health, 28
  letter to Clara, 37
  medal from Ste. Anne de Beaupré for Clara, 73
  visit from Clara, Lou and Mary, 126
St. Patrick's Church, 170
St. Thomas Aquinas School, Ottawa, 9, 46–47
Stewart, Miss (nurse), 63–64
Story of the Royal Ottawa Hospital (1985), xiv
streptomycin, 104–5, 104n18, 116, 133–34, 149
sun lamp treatments, 19

Taylor, Isabel, 220
Temptation Hill, 46–47
Teresa Ann, Sister, 62
thoracoplasty
  Clara's left side, and post-operative course, 36, 38, 43–45, 48–51
  Clara's right side, first one and aftermath, 92–96
  Clara's right side, risks of, 88, 89–91
  Clara's right side, second one and aftermath, 96–99
  description, 17, 36n9
  "shot bag" after thoracoplasty, 50
tubercule bacillus, xii

tuberculosis (TB)
  cases in Canada and worldwide, xiv
  description of disease, xi–xiii
  mortality rate, xiv
  "Sanatorium Age," xiii
  treatment in first half of 20th century, xiii–xiv
tuberculosis throat, 47

V-E Day, 68
V-J Day, 72
Vechter, Max (doctor), 129, 131, 132
Viste, Helen, 37
vital capacity, 48n11

W., Miss (nurse), 155–56, 167–68
Walker, Pearl (nurse), 96, 131, 134
warts, 23, 25
Waxy, Mrs. (nurse), 61–62, 63–66, 70–71
We Have Written (Mary Raina), 225
Wheeze and Sneeze and Shoot the Breeze, vi–vii, xvii
whisper restriction, 47
"white plague," xii
Whitney Building (of the Royal Ottawa), 16, 24(p)
Whitton, Charlotte, 169
whooping cough, 7
Wiese School, Hanna, Alberta, 5, 237
Williamson, Norval (doctor), 221, 223
Winganonimous (toy bear), 67–68, 121, 191
World Health Organization, xiv
World Tuberculosis Day, xv

Yosfvllva, Austria-Hungary, 1